RAIS

HEALTHY

CHILDREN

IN A TOXIC

WORLD

---

101 SMART SOLUTIONS
FOR EVERY FAMILY

Philip J. Landrigan, M.D., Herbert L. Needleman, M.D.,
and Mary Landrigan, M.P.A.

RODALE

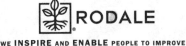

RODALE

WE **INSPIRE** AND **ENABLE** PEOPLE TO IMPROVE
THEIR LIVES AND THE WORLD AROUND THEM

We're always happy to hear from you. For questions or comments concerning the editorial content of this book, please write to:
Rodale Book Readers' Service
33 East Minor Street
Emmaus, PA 18098
Look for other Rodale books wherever books are
sold. Or call us at (800) 848-4735.

For more information about Rodale Organic
Living magazines and books, visit us at
www.organicstyle.com

Editor: Christine Bucks
Cover and Interior Book Designer:
Nancy Smola Biltcliff
Photography Editor: Lyn Horst
Photography Assistant: Jackie L. Ney
Layout Designer: Jennifer H. Giandomenico
Researcher: Diana Erney
Product Specialist: Jodi Schaffer
Indexer: Nanette Bendyna
Editorial Assistance: Claudia Curran and
Susan L. Nickol

Rodale Organic Living Books
Editorial Director: Christopher Hirsheimer
Executive Creative Director: Christin Gangi
Executive Editor: Kathleen DeVanna Fish
Art Director: Patricia Field
Content Assembly Manager: Robert V. Anderson Jr.
Studio Manager: Leslie M. Keefe
Copy Manager: Nancy N. Bailey
Projects Coordinator: Kerrie A. Cadden

**Library of Congress
Cataloging-in-Publication Data**

Landrigan, Philip J.
    Raising healthy children in a toxic world : 101
smart solutions for every family / Philip J. Landrigan,
Herbert L. Needleman, and Mary M. Landrigan.
        p.   cm.
    Includes bibliographical references and index.
    ISBN 0–87596–947–X   paperback
    1. Pediatric toxicology—Popular works.   2. Environ-
mental toxicology—Popular works.   I. Needleman,
Herbert L., 1927-   II. Landrigan, Mary M.   III. Title.
RA1225 .L36 2001
615.9'083—dc21   2001003704

Distributed in the book trade by St. Martin's Press

2 4 6 8 10 9 7 5 3 1   paperback

To our children,
Mary and Jacob, Chris and Clare, and Lizzie;
Sam, Josh, and Yael; and Sara and Stephan.

To their children,
Jonathan Thomas, Erez, Daniella,
Noah, Katherine, and David.

And to their children's children . . .

About the Authors

Philip J. Landrigan, M.D., is professor of pediatrics, Chair of Community and Preventive Medicine, and director of the Center for Children's Health and the Environment at the Mount Sinai School of Medicine. He directed a major study at the National Academy of Sciences on pesticides in children's diets.

Herbert L. Needleman, M.D., is a professor of child psychiatry and pediatrics at the University of Pittsburgh School of Medicine. He is an internationally recognized expert on childhood lead poisoning, and in 1995, in recognition of his research and his advocacy on behalf of children, he was named winner of the prestigious Heinz Award for the Environment.

Mary M. Landrigan, M.P.A., is the director of health education and information for the Westchester County Department of Health in New York. She creates and promotes public health education information on a variety of child and environmental health topics.

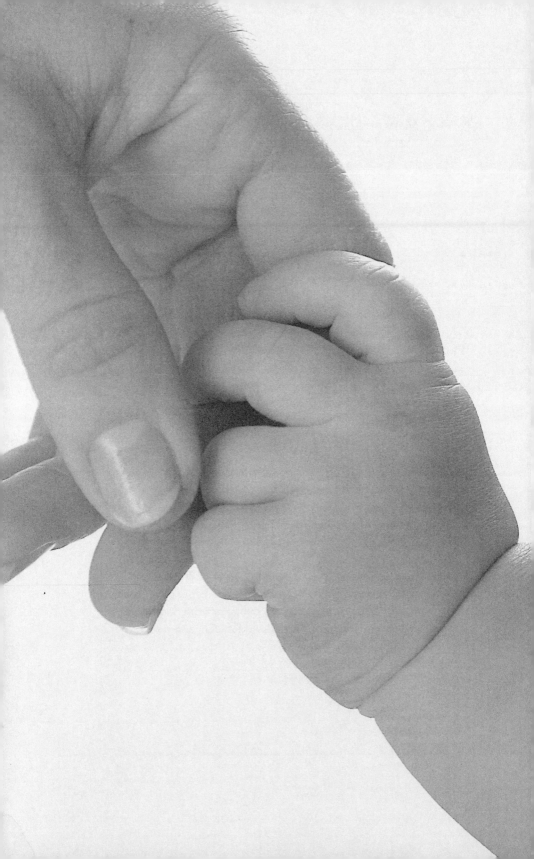

Contents

Acknowledgments

We wish to thank our many friends and colleagues whose advice and inspiration were essential to the creation of this book. We credit our professional colleagues, with whom we work daily to protect children's health from threats in the environment, for their work and their publications toward this vital cause: Mothers and Others for a Livable Planet, whose book *Guide to Natural Baby Care* by Mindy Pennybacker and Aisha Ikramuddin provided incredibly valuable information on natural baby care products and infant care; the Children's Environmental Health Network; Physicians for Social Responsibility; INFORM; the National Religious Partnership for the Environment; and the Children's Health Environmental Coalition (CHEC). CHEC's publication, *The Household Detective*, is an invaluable guide to parents on the lookout for environmental threats to children's health around the home.

We are indebted to Sophie Balk, M.D., F.A.A.P., whose original work in the construction of a household inventory provided a foundation for the environmental checklists presented in this book.

We salute Carol M. Browner, former administrator of the U.S. Environmental Protection Agency, and Ramona Trovato, director of EPA's Office of Children's Health Protection, for their courage and leadership in protecting children's health from environmental threats.

Thanks to Professor Robin Moore, landscape architect at North Carolina State University, for promoting the concept of natural playgrounds.

The table in "Review Those Art Supplies" on page 111 is adapted from "Occupational Hazards in the Arts and Professions" by M. McCann in *Environmental and Occupational Medicine*, William N. Rom, M.D., M.P.H., editor, pages 1206–1207.

Special thanks to our children: Mary F. Landrigan-Ossar, M.D., Ph.D., for her insights and expertise in helping to convert complex scientific and medical information into commonsense tips; Jacob Ossar, Ph.D., for philosophical discussions of ethical concepts in the book; Christopher P. Landrigan, M.D., M.P.H., for providing insight into childhood poisonings from the perspective of an academic pediatrician; Clare L. Landrigan, M.S., for her expertise in child development and her guidance in helping us develop tips for busy parents; Elizabeth M. Landrigan, M.S., for her insight into the geology of water pollution and for her review and editing of the sections on water issues; Samuel Needleman, M.D., for advice about carcinogens; Sara Needleman, L.L.D., for discussions about legal questions; and Joshua Needleman, M.D., for his comments about asthma and air pollution.

We'd also like to thank Nancy Smola Biltcliff for her appealing and easy-to-read design. And last, but far from least, special thanks to our editor at Rodale, Christine Bucks, who shaped the final text and provided insightful questions to help clarify and define our recommendations.

The wisdom and experience are theirs. Any errors or omissions are ours. We thank them all.

Wellfleet, Massachusetts, August 2001

Protecting Your Children

This book is written for you, a parent of a child in today's world.

In today's world, the air we breathe, water we drink, food we eat, homes we live in, and parks where we play are all susceptible to a host of environmental toxins. Although these toxins can affect everyone, those most at risk are our children. Of course, as a parent you want to do everything you can to keep your child safe. But protecting children from environmental toxins may seem like a big challenge.

That's why we wrote this book—to provide you with essential, practical information that you need to protect your child from the numerous environmental toxins that exist in our society.

To make the book easy to follow, we divided it into three parts. The first part focuses on toxins in your home, the second part on toxins in your community, and the third part on ways you can protect yourself from toxins that may affect your reproductive health—and thus your future children. Each part begins with an environmental checklist; you'll need only a few minutes to go through the questions on each checklist. By completing the checklists, you'll find out which environmental toxins are present in your home and community; the accompanying text will tell you just how serious a risk they are for your child and what you can do about them.

In fact, we've provided 101 practical solutions for common environmental toxins such as lead, radon, and pesticides. Some of the solutions consist of changes you can make in your own home, including switching to nontoxic cleaning materials or having your basement tested for radon. Others solutions are ones you can tackle in your child's day care, school, and community.

Environmental health threats are frightening, but you *can* do something about them. Every one of the solutions in this book has proven effective, and all of them are within your reach. So use them to help improve your child's health. The changes you make today can have a profound effect on your child's quality of life—and can pave the way for a healthier environment for future generations.

We wish you success and know it will be yours.

Philip J. Landrigan, M.D.   Herbert L. Needleman, M.D.   Mary M. Landrigan, M.P.A.

PART ONE

PROTECTING YOUR CHILD IN YOUR HOME

AN ENVIRONMENTAL CHECKLIST FOR YOUR HOME

Your home is the focal point of your child's life—it's where he learns to crawl, where he eats and sleeps, where he plays. Home represents a comfortable and safe haven for him . . . yet just how safe is it? Even if your home is brand new, it might not be as safe as you would like to think it is.

To find out what areas of your home might harbor potential environmental hazards, read through this checklist, answering the questions as you go. As you answer, check out the numbers (if any) that follow your responses. Those numbers correspond to the numbered "Smart Solutions" throughout this book that can help you prevent or eliminate the unsafe situation.

LEAD, RADON, AND ASBESTOS

The boxed numbers indicate which SMART SOLUTION(s) you should review.

How OLD is your house?
○ built before 1970 [1] [19] [21] [23] [55] [56]
○ built after 1970 [1] [2] [13] [51] [55] [57]

Is there chipping or peeling PAINT
in your house?
○ Yes [19] [20] [21] [22] [24] [25]   ○ No

Is there chipping and peeling PAINT on the windowsills?
○ Yes [19] [21] [24]   ○ No

Do the WINDOW WELLS have solid material?
○ Yes   ○ No [19]

Is the PLUMBING more than 40 years old?
○ Yes [23] [24]   ○ No

(continued)

The boxed numbers indicate which SMART SOLUTION(s) you should review.

Is the PLUMBING less than 5 years old?
○ Yes   ○ No 23

Do you have LEAD PIPES?
○ Yes 23 24   ○ No

Has your water been tested for LEAD?
○ Yes   ○ No 23 24

Do you have a BASEMENT?
○ Yes 48 51 52 55 56 57
○ No

Are the basement PIPES insulated?
○ Yes 56 57   ○ No

Are any CEILINGS covered with sprayed-on or troweled-on material?
○ Yes 56 57   ○ No

Are there SLEEPING or PLAYING areas in the basement?
○ Yes 55   ○ No

Are there CRACKS in the basement floor or walls or GAPS between the basement ceiling and walls?
○ Yes 55   ○ No

HEATING AND AIR QUALITY CONCERNS

Do you have one or more working FIREPLACES? Does SMOKE enter the room when you use the fireplace?
○ Yes 17   ○ No

If you have a WOOD-BURNING STOVE in your home, is it properly vented?
○ Yes   ○ No 15

Do you have STORM WINDOWS?
○ Yes 16 17   ○ No

Do you have a GAS STOVE?
○ Yes 15   ○ No

Does your gas stove have a PILOT LIGHT?
○ Yes 15   ○ No

Do you use your gas stove for HEAT?
○ Yes 15   ○ No

Do you use KEROSENE space heaters?
○ Yes 15   ○ No

Do you use a gas CLOTHES DRYER?
○ Yes 15   ○ No

Do you have forced HOT-AIR heat?
○ Yes 15   ○ No

Do you have an electronic AIR CLEANER?
○ Yes 17   ○ No

Do you have a furnace HUMIDIFIER?
○ Yes 12   ○ No

Is your home INSULATED?
○ Yes 57   ○ No

PESTICIDES AND OTHER HARMFUL PRODUCTS

Has your house ever been treated for TERMITES?
○ Yes 31   ○ No

Do you know what PESTICIDE was used during the termite treatment?
○ Yes   ○ No 31

Do you use PESTICIDES on your lawn or garden?
○ Yes 29 30 32 33 34 44
○ No

Do you use a commercial LAWN SERVICE?
○ Yes 34   ○ No

Do you STORE pesticides in the house?
○ Yes 30 32 52   ○ No

Do you DISPOSE of unused or leftover pesticides at a hazardous waste facility?
○ Yes   ○ No 52

Do you keep old PRESCRIPTION DRUGS in the medicine cabinet?
○ Yes 46 52   ○ No

Do you keep MOTOR OIL or GASOLINE in the house or garage?
○ Yes 52   ○ No

Do you keep SOLVENTS such as alcohol, toluene, dry-cleaning fluids, or degreasing solvents in the house?
○ Yes 17 52   ○ No

Does anyone in your house SMOKE?
○ Yes 3 15   ○ No

Does anyone in your household MAKE stained glass, pottery, jewelry, or fishing weights?
○ Yes 24   ○ No

Does anyone REFINISH furniture at your home?
○ Yes 54   ○ No

Do you use any of the following PRODUCTS: toilet-bowl cleaners, room deodorizers, polishes, varnishes, or paint thinners?
○ Yes 17 47 48 49 51   ○ No

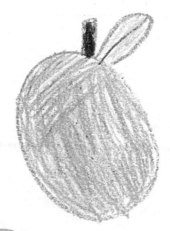

8 Special Concerns for Your Baby's Room

YOU MAY already have a vision of what you want your baby's room to look like. Perhaps you see soft pastel walls accented with a border of stars and the moon—or brighter reds, blues, yellows, and greens with a farm animal theme. No matter what you choose for the decor, though, you know you want your baby's room to be as comfortable and soothing as possible.

You may also have certain ideas about the types of products you want to use on your baby, such as shampoos, wipes, soaps, and powders. After all, there are almost as many baby-care products available on the market as there are personal-care products for moms and dads, so you have plenty to choose from.

But while a cute room and a sweet-smelling baby paint a nice picture, what you really need to keep in mind is your baby's health. Your baby's room should be a place where you're not exposing him to toxins, and the products you apply to his tiny body should be harmless, as well. Common items such as overstuffed furniture, fragrant baby soap, and talcum powder may seem safe enough, but in reality they're potential hazards that may affect your child's health. To help you avoid those hazards, we've put together the following guidelines so you can create the best possible conditions for your baby's room—and choose the least-toxic baby-care products.

1 SMART SOLUTION
Renovate the baby's room well before you're ready to start a family.

Because of all the possible toxins the developing fetus or baby could be exposed to, avoid household renovations during pregnancy or when your child is an infant. As soon as you decide it's time to start a family—even before the baby has been conceived—consider doing any renovations to the room that will become the baby's room. To help you with your renovations, we've come up with this handy checklist to alert you to potential problem areas, with hints for solving the problems following the checklist. (The checklist is in order of importance, starting with the things you should be most concerned about.)

☆☆
Important

△
Easy

☐ Peeling or chipping paint

☐ Dirty or dull paint on walls

☐ Problems with insects or rodents

☐ Wall-to-wall carpet

☐ Dampness or mold

☐ Worn wooden or vinyl floors

☐ Windows that won't open

☐ Old wallpaper

☐ Overstuffed furniture

☐ Heavy curtains

Peeling and chipping paint. Peeling and chipping lead-based paint is the number-one source of childhood lead poisoning. (See Smart Solutions 19–22) Infants are particularly susceptible to lead because it can damage their developing brains and nervous systems.

The first step to take when you see peeling or chipping paint in the baby's room (or elsewhere in the house) is to have the paint tested by a certified lead paint inspector or certified laboratory. To find a certified inspector or laboratory, check with your state or city health department or with the regional office of the Environmental Protection Agency. Check with the inspector or lab to make sure the inspection will be done with an XRF (X-ray fluorescence) detector, not with the crayon-type detectors often sold in hardware stores. (See 19 20 for more information on lead testing, including why the XRF is better than a crayon-type detector.)

If you do have lead paint in the baby's room, enlist expert guidance on what to do next. Call your state health department to find out what local resources are available to help you with lead paint abatement (removal). Don't attempt to remove the lead paint yourself without expert guidance; in fact, it's best to have the job done by an experienced, trained, certified lead paint abatement contractor. For more information on removing lead paint properly, check out *Reducing Lead Hazards When Remodeling Your Home* (see "Recommended Reading" on page 144) and the Alliance to End Childhood Lead Poisoning at www.aeclp.org.

We realize that you may need to do other renovations in the baby's room before the lead paint is removed. Just be extremely careful not to sand lead paint, and don't clean up any paint chips using a household vacuum. These methods pulverize the lead paint, dispersing it as dust throughout the house.

Dull or dirty paint on walls. If you're going to want a new, clean, shiny painted room for your baby, paint it now. (We are assuming that you have already had your house tested for lead paint and have corrected any lead paint problems; see "Peeling and chipping paint" on page 5 and 19 – 22 for more information on lead paint abatement.)

When choosing paint, buy the least-toxic paint available. (See 53) Water-based latex paint has fewer toxic volatile organic compounds (VOCs) than oil-based paint. Keep in mind, though, that even the least-toxic paints will release VOCs into the room for days or weeks after painting. You don't want a pregnant mom or a new baby inhaling unnecessary indoor pollutants. The best way to deal with VOCs, aside from avoiding them in the first place, is to thoroughly air out the room for a week or so after painting. Also, absolutely avoid paints that contain mercury compounds as fungicides. These are often sold as "bathroom paint" or "kitchen paint." Mercury is a toxic metal that can damage a person's nervous system and brain—and can be emitted as the paint dries.

VOCs (VOLATILE ORGANIC COMPOUNDS) FROM PAINT CAN HANG AROUND FOR MONTHS IN A CLOSED SPACE. TO AVOID THIS, AIR OUT A ROOM WELL—RIGHT AFTER PAINTING IT.

Problems with insects or rodents. If you've been having trouble with pest insects or rodents, now is the time to nip those problems in the bud—nontoxically, of course. (See 29 – 34 for information on just how to do that.)

Wall-to-wall carpeting. If you have wall-to-wall carpeting in the baby's room, you may want to remove it since it's a potential dust collector and a haven for molds, fungi, and other respiratory irritants. Carpet shampoos aren't a big help, either, as some of them can also irritate the respiratory system. (See 13)

Replacing old wall-to-wall carpeting with new synthetic wall-to-wall carpeting isn't your best option. New carpeting, like new furniture and new paint, can emit formaldehyde, a cancer-causing chemical, and VOCs that can pollute the air in the baby's room and in the house. These VOCs can build up, especially if you have many new pieces of furniture, new carpeting, or freshly painted walls in the house. The noticeable "new carpet" or "new furniture" smell is a good indication that VOCs are being emitted. The problem with VOCs is that they can be respiratory irritants and cause your eyes to itch and burn. Some VOCs can cause more serious health effects, such as interference with brain function and slowed reflexes (if levels are high enough in the room or house). New babies don't need that aggravation—and neither do moms-to-be! The best solution is to replace the wall-to-wall carpeting with area rugs that you can shake out or wash on a regular basis.

Dampness or mold. A damp or musty-smelling room may be an indication that water is getting into walls, ceilings, or floors from a leaky roof or leaky windows. And damp walls and ceilings can host a variety of molds and fungi that can trigger allergies or other health problems. You can partially fix the situation by installing a dehumidifier. However, a dehumidifier needs careful and regular maintenance, including emptying and cleaning, to avoid buildup of harmful bacteria, molds, or fungi in the machine itself. The best remedy for a damp or musty room is to figure out and permanently fix the cause of the problem.

Worn wooden or vinyl floors. Wooden floors that have lost their finish can absorb liquids and then slowly decay. Worn vinyl floors can allow liquids to seep through the finish or through the seams onto the floor base. Both of these situations can lead to the growth of mold and fungus. If you have worn wooden floors, you should refinish them. Keep in mind, though, that synthetic polyurethanes and varnishes release chemical irritants into the room for days or weeks after the floor has been refinished. These VOCs can cause respiratory irritation and other health problems, particularly if the room or house is closed up. So if you're going to refinish the floors, do it before you have a pregnant mom, a new baby, or a toddler in the house.

If there is an existing wooden floor underneath your worn vinyl floor, you can simply remove the vinyl to expose the wood. Or, you can tear out the old vinyl and install new vinyl. Just make sure you air out the room after installing the vinyl—until you no longer smell the new "plastic" smell that lets you know the vinyl flooring is emitting VOCs.

Windows that won't open. Windows that won't open can be a symptom of a moisture problem that needs correction (see the previous point about dampness). Or, they could simply be painted shut. If the windows are painted with lead paint, you'll need to be careful when trying to get them open. If you don't take proper precautions, you could create a lead paint hazard. (See 19–22) Any way you look at it, you'll want to be able to open your windows easily to air out the baby's room, so fix them now.

Old wallpaper. If you have faded, outdated wallpaper covering the baby's room, you might decide to update the look with new wallpaper. Today's wallpapers are often made with or coated with synthetic plastics, though, and the adhesives that affix them to the walls are also synthetic plastics that emit vapors as they dry. The smell of a newly wallpapered room reminds you that VOCs are being emitted, so wallpaper and ventilate the room well before a pregnant mom or new infant is in the house.

Overstuffed furniture. Overstuffed furniture may be extremely comfortable, but it collects dust and can be a source of dust mites and allergens. (See 10 12) If you decide to keep a rocking chair with an overstuffed cushion in the room, try minimizing the dust problem by covering the cushion with the new allergen-barrier fabrics being sold as pillowcase covers or mattress covers, then put a zippered slipcover over that. Since new fabric can also be a source of indoor air pollutants, choose washable fabric and launder it first.

Heavy curtains. How often do you take down those heavy drapes for a good cleaning? Probably not too often, just because doing so is a chore. The longer between cleanings, however, the more dust and pollen (which are respiratory irritants) the drapes collect. So replace them with washable, lightweight fabric curtains. (See 9) By using washable curtains, you can throw them in the washing machine on a regular basis to get rid of the dust and pollen—plus, you'll save on dry-cleaning bills. You'll also avoid the potential release of toxic dry-cleaning chemicals (perchlorethylene or trichloroethylene) into the baby's room after the drapes are cleaned.

2 SMART SOLUTION
Use "prudent avoidance" with regard to EMFs.

☆☆
Important

△△
Moderately Easy

An electromagnetic field (EMF) is an invisible but measurable field created when electricity flows along an electrical wire. These fields vary in strength and size, from turning on an appliance to the power sent along the lines to businesses and homes in your community. The strongest fields surround high-tension power lines—the large overhead lines that can carry electricity long distances from the electric utility plant to smaller lines. The strength of an EMF diminishes rapidly as you move away from the source of the field. Over 3 feet from an EMF created by a household appliance, the EMF level significantly diminishes. For high-tension power lines, the EMFs don't drop off until around 100 yards, or the length of a football field.

The concern over EMFs is that some studies indicate they cause childhood health problems. For example:

- In 1979, two American researchers in Denver reviewed childhood cancer in relation to the proximity of the children's homes to power lines. They found that children who had died from cancer were twice as likely to have lived within 131 feet of a high current power line than other children studied. Because high electrical currents generate large EMFs, they attributed the increase in childhood cancer to the EMFs.

- In 1993, Swedish researchers found that children exposed to electromagnetic radiation from high-tension lines were twice as likely to have leukemia as children not exposed to such radiation. (The fact that researchers in Sweden have access to information to document a child's exposure to EMFs over a lifetime makes this study very well designed.) The children were all under 15 years old; those who developed leukemia had been exposed to the radiation for at least 2 years.

- In 1999, a Canadian study of children's exposure to EMFs from high-tension lines found that those who had been exposed for at least 2 years had an elevated risk of leukemia. The study also showed that children under the age of 6 years who were exposed to EMFs from high-tension lines were almost six times as likely to develop leukemia than other children in the same age group who didn't live near high-tension lines.

EMFS IN YOUR HOME

HERE ARE some examples of the size of electromagnetic fields (EMFs) caused by common household appliances.

Magnetic Fields (mG) at Indicated Approximate Distances

HOUSEHOLD APPLIANCE	1 INCH	6 INCHES	1 FOOT	2 FEET	3 FEET	4 FEET
Television*	25–5,000	—	4–20	—	0.1–2.0	—
Fluorescent light*	400–4,000	—	5–20	—	0.1–3.0	—
Microwave oven*	750–2,000	—	40–80	—	3.0–8.0	—
Electric cookstove*	60–2,000	—	4–40	—	0.1–1.0	—
Can opener†	—	500–1,500	40–300	3–30	—	0–4
Clothes washer*	8–400	—	2–30	—	0.1–2.0	—
Portable heater†	—	5–150	1–40	0–8	—	0–1
Blender†	—	30–100	5–20	0–3	—	0
Dishwasher†	—	10–100	6–30	2–7	—	0–1
Conventional clock†	—	1–30	2–5	0–3	—	—
Baby monitor†	—	—	4–15	0–2	—	—
Coffeemaker†	—	4–10	0–1	0	—	0
Digital clock†	—	0–8	0–2	0–1	—	—

*Source: "Electric and Magnetic Fields,"
www.hsph.harvard.edu/Organizations/Canprevent/emf.html
†Source: EMFs in Your Environment, EPA, 1992

Because scientists continue to find links between EMFs and childhood cancers, we recommend that you adopt a habit of "prudent avoidance"—meaning you should do what you can to adjust your lifestyle so you avoid this suspected health risk. Here are some prudent things you may want to do to avoid EMFs.

- Avoid buying a home underneath high-tension electrical wires or within 100 yards of a major transformer.

- Position the baby's crib as far as possible from the corner of the house where the electricity comes into the house from outside lines.

- Place any electric appliances, including clocks, across the room from where the baby sleeps rather than right beside the baby's crib.

- Use a baby monitor that's sensitive enough to be placed a few feet away from the baby to minimize the baby's exposure to EMFs from the monitor.

- Keep the baby (and you) at least 3 feet away from televisions, microwave ovens, and other electrical household appliances when they are in use.

- Avoid spending time with the baby in areas close to high-tension wires.

- Avoid using electric blankets in the crib.

A fundamental difference in assessing the hazard posed by high-tension lines and most appliances has to do with duration of exposure. You usually turn appliances on for only brief periods of time, whereas EMFs from high-tension lines are present 24 hours a day, 7 days a week.

3 SMART SOLUTION
Don't smoke in the baby's room.

One of the most important things you can do for the health of your baby is to make sure the air in her room is fresh and clean. And that means absolutely no smoking in her room. (Of course, no smoking anywhere in the house is an even better policy to follow.)

☆☆☆
Very
Important

△
Easy

Exposure to secondhand smoke (i.e., "used" smoke that's already been exhaled from someone else's lungs, or "sidestream" smoke that drifts across the room from someone's burning cigarette) can be very harmful to your baby's health—and to your health, as well. Secondhand smoke contains known cancer-causing chemicals, meaning when you or a family member smoke, your baby is being exposed to those bad chemicals, too. As you begin to think about bringing a new life into this world, do everything you can to make it a healthy life. Ultimately, that means stopping smoking.

This is not the only time we will warn you of the dangers of smoking. According to the American Cancer Society, tobacco claims more than 400,000 lives in the United States every year. About half of the smokers between 35 and 69 years of age die prematurely—losing up to 25 years of their normal lifespan. Putting out that last cigarette may be the most important step you can take to add up to 25 years to your life. So take that step today.

SMART SOLUTION

4 Install a smoke detector in the baby's room.

Of course you know that a smoke detector can save your family's lives from a fire in your home. But it can also save you and your family from exposure to the potentially fatal, toxic by-products of smoke from burning synthetics and plastics that are so much a part of today's households. So in addition to the baby's room, make sure to place smoke detectors in each person's bedroom and at the top of every stairway.

☆☆☆
Very
Important

△
Easy

(*Note:* Use care when handling and discarding smoke detectors. Smoke detectors use minute quantities of radioactive materials to sense the presence of combustion in an area. To avoid being exposed to the radioactive material, discard according to the directions given with the smoke detector or call your municipality or fire department to find out if they have any preferred method of disposal.)

To get an idea of the different types of toxic materials that are produced when household items burn, take a look at the following chart.

SYNTHETIC MATERIAL	FOUND IN	TOXIN PRODUCED WHEN BURNED AND ITS EFFECT
Vinyl plastics	Toys, household items	Dioxin; cancer
Acrylonitriles	Lucite plastics, such as paperweights and clipboards	Hydrogen cyanide; death by asphyxiation
Polyurethanes	Chair cushions, insulation	Toluene di-isocyanate; asthma
Vinyl chloride	Plastic toys and furnishings	Hydrochloric acid; respiratory irritation
All of the above	All of the above	Carbon monoxide; asphyxiation

Also keep in mind that you should check all of your smoke detectors twice a year to make sure the batteries are working properly. (A good time to check them is in the spring and fall, when you adjust your clocks for Daylight Savings Time.) Follow the manufacturer's directions regarding the number and type of batteries to be used in the smoke detectors, as well as the directions for installing your smoke detectors properly.

5

SMART SOLUTION

Choose nontoxic baby shampoos, detergents, ointments, and wipes.

In their book *Natural Baby Care*, authors Mindy Pennybacker and Aisha Ikramuddin identify a wealth of nontoxic and environmentally friendly ways to take care of your new baby. Some of their suggestions for baby-care products that are safe and natural are listed here.

☆
Good Idea

△
Easy

Baby soap. The best soap for baby is no soap at all: just plain warm water and a washcloth. This should suffice during the "mild dribbles and drool" stage, the authors note. For those situations where plain warm water may not suffice (for example, if your baby is a chronic spitter of milk or formula), use a mild soap such as Dove or an olive-oil castile soap for cleanups. (See "Resources" on page 145.) When baby begins to crawl around the floor and get into real dirt, Dove, an olive-oil castile soap, or an unscented, nonadditive "baby" soap are good ideas. Avoid choosing products that have fragrances or additives that make bubbles. Fragrances can cause sensitivities in baby's skin; additives that make bubbles can make the baby more prone to urinary tract infections.

Baby shampoos. Stick with fragrance-free baby shampoos as opposed to adult shampoos, which are too harsh for baby. However, the authors of *Natural Baby Care* suggest you try the "no tears" variety on yourself to be sure that it will actually produce "no tears" for baby.

Detergents. Mild is the key word when it comes to detergents for baby because his skin is so sensitive. Many pediatricians recommend detergents (such as Dreft) designed specifically for infant laundry. Babies with sensitive skin will benefit from the use of mild detergent, at least as long as they are in diapers. Check with your pediatrician to find out how long you should keep separating baby clothes from the rest of the family laundry.

Diaper rash ointments. A general rule of thumb is to avoid ointments that have a long list of ingredients on the package. The more ingredients, the more likely the baby is going to be sensitive to one of them. Ointments that contain primarily zinc oxide are the best choice for preventing and treating diaper rash. You can also use petroleum jelly to protect baby's skin.

ADDED FRAGRANCES IN DISPOSABLE DIAPERS MAY CAUSE AN ALLERGIC REACTION IN SOME BABIES. THE PLASTIC COVERS MAY ALSO PROMOTE DIAPER RASH.

Wipes. Commercial baby wipes contain alcohol and other ingredients that can irritate a baby's skin. A good alternative to commercial wipes is room temperature or warm water on a plain cotton wipe. To avoid running to the sink for water every time your baby needs a diaper change, try this helpful hint: Fill a plastic squirt bottle with 1 cup of water and 1 teaspoon of baking soda and keep it handy for quick cleanups. Change any unused solution weekly.

6 SMART SOLUTION
Avoid routinely using antibacterial cleaners.

Antibacterial cleaners seem like such a good idea—after all, they must get rid of germs—and who's not for that?

☆☆
Important

But you need to step back for a moment and think about what you're doing when you kill germs. Although some microbes cause disease, many are helpful and even necessary to our survival. For example, the normal functioning of your digestive system relies on the presence of the beneficial bacteria that live in your intestinal tract. And if you've ever taken antibiotics, you've probably experienced the discomfort of diarrhea or a runaway yeast infection—the impact of the temporary disruption of the normal bacteria in your body. When you kill off the normal beneficial bacteria with antibiotics, less desirable bacteria and yeast can grow.

△
Easy

So what happens when you use antibacterial cleaners? The usual sea of microbes in the environment is temporarily disrupted. You kill the weakest germs, giving the survivors free reign to multiply and fill the void. If those stronger germs are pathogenic (the type that cause disease), you've just enabled more toxic germs to inhabit the area you've cleaned—the baby's room. So, by killing the good germs and allowing the bad germs to flourish, you expose the baby to more (and stronger), not fewer, germs and sicknesses.

Instead of using antibacterial products for routine cleanup, use soap and water. To disinfect areas contaminated during a serious illness, try a solution of chlorine bleach in water (about ¼ cup of household bleach to 1 gallon of water). This mild solution is also perfect for cleaning up spills and disinfecting laundry. (Before using the solution, test a small area to make sure it doesn't damage the fabric or surface you're going to apply it to, and make sure to let the fumes dissipate before allowing the baby back into the area.)

7 SMART SOLUTION
Skip the talcum powder.

Who can resist the sweet smell of baby's skin, lightly powdered after a bath? But powder is one thing to keep out of baby's room and off of baby. In reality, powder can cause some pretty severe health problems, such as pneumonia and lung inflammation, when the baby inhales it. Many powders contain particles of talc, a mineral that is a component of talcum powder and that's also a close cousin of the dangerous mineral asbestos.

Bottom line (no pun intended!): Keep all powders, as well as cornstarch (which can cause choking if inhaled by baby), out of baby's room and breathing range.

☆
Good
Idea

△
Easy

8 SMART SOLUTION
Use silicone nipples and pacifiers.

Baby bottle nipples and pacifiers made of polyvinyl chloride (PVC) or other plastics can leach potentially harmful chemicals known as phthalates, which are used to keep the nipples soft. Phthalates are suspected of being endocrine disrupters—chemicals that mimic normal body hormones and may possibly interfere with normal body functions. Some phthalates have also been found to increase a person's risk of cancer. While research on endocrine disrupters is still in its infancy, we think it wise to avoid exposing your baby to endocrine disrupters whenever possible. And that means using silicone nipples and pacifiers instead of plastic or latex rubber ones.

☆☆
Important

△
Easy

BANNING PVCS

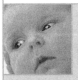

SOME EUROPEAN countries are in various stages of banning the production and sale of polyvinyl chloride (PVC) baby toys that contain phthalates because of their potential health risks. These include Germany, Sweden, Norway, Denmark, Italy, Greece, Finland, and Austria.

The U.S. Consumer Product Safety Commission has recommended voluntary action by the toy industry to remove phthalates from their products—and we endorse that recommendation. Some manufacturers of PVC-free toys in the United States include Brio, Early Start, LEGO, Little Tykes, Primetime Playthings, and Sassy Products.

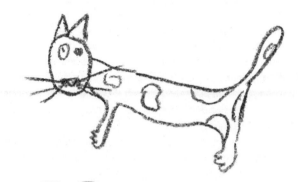

10 Ways to Avoid Allergy and Asthma Attacks

YOUR CHILDREN are more vulnerable to harm from air pollutants than you are. And that harm can come in the form of allergies, asthma, or both.

Allergies are overly sensitive bodily responses to exposure to any number of trigger substances called allergens. Allergies frequently appear in children whose other family members have a history of allergies. The allergy or bodily response may be as mild as itchy eyes, a runny nose, and sneezing— or as severe as asthma. Some allergies, such as those from peanuts, can even be life threatening. (See Smart Solution 42) Common allergens include plant pollens, dust mites, molds, and some foods. In this section, we will discuss those allergens that cause respiratory system distress, such as dust mites.

Asthma is a breathing disorder whose symptoms include wheezing, coughing, difficulty breathing, and chest tightness. It's caused by inflammation and spasms of a person's airway. Asthma is epidemic in the United States. In 1993, there were about 275 asthma hospitalizations for every 100,000 children under the age of 14; in 1995, that number rose to 396.

Asthma has both a genetic and an environmental component. Ken Olden, Ph.D., director of the National Institute of Environmental Health Science has described the situation as genetics loading the gun and environmental factors pulling the trigger. From a genetic standpoint, children whose mothers or fathers had asthma as a child are more likely to have asthma than those whose parents had no history of asthma. The environmental component is equally compelling. Children whose mothers or fathers smoke during pregnancy or during the first few years of their lives are more likely to have asthma than those whose parents didn't smoke.

Research also shows that repeated exposure to substances in the environment that produce allergies can cause a child's airway to become inflamed and react more severely each time that child is exposed to an allergen. Some of the most potent allergens associated with asthma attacks in children are tobacco smoke, dust mites, cockroaches, and furry animals.

But these environmental components—of both allergies and asthma—are things that you can do something about. Some changes are easy to make, while others may alter your family's lifestyle in a significant way. We suggest you carefully examine each room in your house and consider making the changes we suggest. Before tackling some of the larger lifestyle issues (such as finding a new home for your indoor pet), you may want to talk it over with your own pediatrician or health-care provider to see what's best for your child. The recommendations in this book are meant as guidelines, not as hard-and-fast rules to be followed without thought.

Because children have a lifetime ahead of them, they have more opportunity to develop diseases that are a result

WHY AIR POLLUTANTS HARM KIDS

THE EFFECTS of air pollution can take a harder toll on your children than on you for three main reasons.

First, children's airways are small in diameter, meaning a pollutant that only slightly irritates an adult's airway will significantly irritate and narrow the airway of a child. And that can produce wheezing, reactive airway disease (hypersensitivity to allergens), or asthma.

Second, because children are more active and have much more active metabolisms than adults, they take in more air relative to their size than adults do. They breathe more rapidly and inhale more pollutants per pound of body weight.

And third, children's lungs are still growing (their lungs don't reach maturity until about age 20). Repeated exposure to air pollution and repeated bouts of asthma can limit the growth of a child's lungs and predispose her to chronic lung disease.

of early exposure to air pollution. Repeated bouts of severe asthma can lead to lifelong respiratory problems. To help nip those potential problems in the bud, here are ten practical ways to minimize air pollutants and allergens in your home—and help your kids breathe easier.

9 SMART SOLUTION
Lighten up on the curtains.

Curtains can collect an amazing amount of dust. When dirt that's tracked into your house on muddy boots and soccer shoes dries, it becomes airborne and finds its way onto the curtains. Pollen from grass and trees that's tracked indoors also ends up on your curtains, as well as dust released from overstuffed furniture when your kids use it as an indoor jungle gym.

☆☆☆
Very
Important

△
Easy

Heavy drapes or curtains made of dry-clean-only fabric are usually the worst dust collectors because they're expensive to have professionally laundered. It can be tempting to leave them up for months—or even years—between cleanings.

To combat dusty curtains, your best bet is to replace all dry-clean-only types with machine-washable curtains. (This may seem like a big expense, but it really will decrease the amount of dust in your home. Plus, you'll save money by not having to pay to have them dry-cleaned.) You might even want to try a different look, with light curtains topped with a valance or swag that you can easily take down for cleaning. Once you have machine-washable curtains up, be sure to wash them at least four times a year.

10 SMART SOLUTION
Cover up mattresses, box springs, and pillows.

Pillows, mattresses, box springs, sheets, and blankets are all home to dust mites—microscopic creatures that trigger allergies in kids. While you can wash sheets and blankets (and should do so on a weekly basis), you can't exactly stuff a mattress into the washing machine.

☆☆☆
Very
Important

Easy

What you can do, though, is cover your child's mattress and box spring with zippered plastic covers (you can find them in department and bed-and-bath stores). Before you buy any covers, crumple them to see how quiet they are. Some types are made of plastic that stays soft and quiet to the touch, while other types are made of plastic that crackles. Never use thin plastic, such as the plastic that comes with dry cleaning. It can get wrapped around a child's face and become a safety hazard.

Make sure you buy a cover that completely encloses the mattress. It's easy to find mattress covers that are made like fitted sheets, with elastic around the edges, but resist the urge to settle for those. They don't do the job because they don't completely enclose the mattress top and bottom. Once you get your mattress cover home, wash it before putting the mattress into it to get rid of that "plastic" smell.

You should also cover your child's pillow with the same type of plastic before putting the pillow in the pillowcase. Always check with your pediatrician about using a plastic pillow or mattress cover, though, before you actually buy one. A child who drools or sweats when sleeping may develop a rash because the plastic cover may trap moisture, causing skin irritation.

SMART SOLUTION
11 Choose stuffed animals wisely.

In addition to invading your pillows and blankets, dust mites also make their home within the fur of all of those stuffed animals your kids love to snuggle. If your child has significant allergies or any type of wheezing or asthma, non-washable stuffed animals should be off-limits. Dusty stuffed animals can trigger an asthma attack or cause uncomfortable allergy symptoms, such as a runny nose and itchy eyes. And any time your child is exposed to those dusty stuffed animals, his asthma or wheezing can actually become worse or more chronic. If you want your child to breathe easy, make sure that any stuffed animals he owns are washable—and then throw them in the washing machine once a week. After all, if your child can't breathe, nothing else matters.

☆☆
Important

△△
Moderately
Easy

If your child doesn't have allergies or has only rare bouts of milder allergies and no regular bouts of wheezing, you can be a bit more lenient about letting him have nonwashable stuffed animals. However, you should be aware that the dust in the stuffed animals might be contributing to your child's occasional misery. And continual exposure to allergens can make a mild case of allergies worse. If your child's bouts with allergies increase or he starts wheezing more often, you should reconsider your decision to let him have nonwashable stuffed animals.

Here are a few other hints to keep in mind with regard to nonwashable stuffed animals.

- Give the animals a "vacation" when your child has a cold or seems particularly allergy-prone. Put the animals in a plastic bag in another room, and give your child a few washable stuffed animals to play with. If your child's symptoms redevelop when you give the stuffed animals back, consider phasing out the nonwashable stuffed animals. Move most of them out of the child's room while you make the transition from nonwashable stuffed animals to washable ones.

- Don't keep hordes of stuffed animals on your child's bed or stashed in his room.

- Try frequently vacuuming the stuffed animals to decrease the number of dust mites.

- Dust mites like normal household temperatures and humidity. To reduce their humidity and raise their temperature, tumble the stuffed animals in your clothes dryer weekly. Check with the manufacturer beforehand to make sure you won't ruin the toys.

12 SMART SOLUTION
Stay ahead of dust bunnies.

Those wispy, pesky balls of dust that crop up under beds and behind furniture also contribute their fair share to respiratory problems. The easiest way to beat dust bunnies is to clean rooms weekly with a dusting tool designed to collect the dust, not just push it around.

☆ Good Idea

You might also want to invest in a vacuum cleaner with a HEPA (high-efficiency particulate air) filter. HEPA filters are industry-grade filters designed to meet certain air pollution standards: Vacuums with HEPA filters don't just redistribute dust into the room air, as some vacuums without HEPA filters do. If you use a vacuum with a HEPA filter, you'll be certain to send clean air—not just more dust—back into the room when you clean.

 Easy

A room humidifier or a humidifier that attaches to your furnace is another option you can use to help decrease those dust bunnies. If you choose to use a humidifier, whether it's one for a room or a furnace attachment, take these simple precautions to prevent the buildup of mildew and mold, which can increase allergy symptoms.

Change the water frequently. If you have a small, portable, or tabletop humidifier, empty and clean it daily with a mild detergent to avoid mildew buildup and bacteria growth. If the humidifier has already developed mold or mildew, soak a cloth in a solution of chlorine bleach in water (a scant ¼ cup to 1 gallon of water) and wipe down the humidifier inside and out.

Keep the filters clean. If your humidifier has permanent filters, make sure to clean them regularly. Change disposable filters on a regular basis.

Stay on top of hygiene. If you have a larger or more permanent humidifier or a furnace humidifier, empty the container every 2 weeks and clean it with a mild solution of detergent and water or, if the manufacturer's instructions allow, use a mild solution of chlorine bleach and water.

Make sure that your humidifier keeps the room at less than 50 percent humidity since dust mites thrive once the humidity level is over 50 percent. If your humidifier doesn't have a gauge to measure humidity, you can buy one at your local hardware store.

13 SMART SOLUTION
Get rid of wall-to-wall carpeting.

Wall-to-wall carpeting can generate lots of problems, from cradle to grave. New carpeting emits chemicals, such as formaldehyde, that are respiratory irritants. As new carpeting ages, it collects dust, which can trigger allergies and asthma. The inevitable coffee and juice spills encourage mold to grow in the carpeting, which can cause everything from sneezing and eye irritation to shortness of breath.

☆☆
Important

△△
Moderately
Easy

You might think that shampooing your carpet would eliminate those problems. But rug shampoos aren't the answer because they contain toxic respiratory irritants. When shampooed carpet dries, the shampoo residue (containing the toxic irritants) becomes airborne. Once inhaled, the residue can cause shortness of breath and wheezing. In fact, studies by the National Institute for Occupational Safety and Health have shown that ingredients in rug shampoos cause respiratory irritation and allergy symptoms such as watering eyes.

If you have wall-to-wall carpeting in your house, your best option is to replace all of it with machine-washable cotton or synthetic rugs. If you can replace only some of the wall-to-wall carpeting, start with your child's room first.

Of course, replacing the carpeting may not be an option for you. In that case, frequently vacuum the carpet and establish a "no food or drink" rule in rooms with carpet. Air out the house often (see Smart Solution 16), especially on those bright, dry days when the wind blows briskly through the house. And instead of using regular rug shampoos, try environmentally friendly products (see "Resources" on page 145).

14 SMART SOLUTION
Choose a pet that doesn't shed.

☆☆ Important

△△△ Difficult

Dogs and cats shed fur and dander, both potent allergens. If your child has significant allergies or any type of wheezing or asthma, you shouldn't have a furry pet that lives indoors or comes into the house. Animal dander can trigger an asthma attack or cause uncomfortable allergy symptoms such as a runny nose and itchy eyes. We strongly advise you to put your child's ability to breathe freely ahead of her (or your) fondness for furry pets.

If you must have a dog, keep it outside. Letting Fido in the house, even some of the time, will result in dander and allergens in your home, too. Of course, you might already have a dog—or a cat—that lives indoors. In this case, you'll need to find a new home for your beloved pet if your child has asthma or allergies. We empathize with you if you must find a new home for your pet (or exclude it from your living quarters), but the ability of your child to breathe freely is more important. The best solution may be to find a neighbor or relative who lives close by who will keep the pet, and let your child visit the pet (outdoors) on a regular basis.

Better pet choices for a child with allergies or asthma include birds and fish. Avoid reptiles such as snakes, lizards, turtles, and iguanas, though. They carry salmonella, a bacterium that causes a severe gastrointestinal illness and that can be life threatening to infants.

If your child doesn't have allergies and has only rare bouts of milder allergies and no regular bouts of wheezing, you don't have to be as stringent about allowing furry pets indoors. However, keep in mind that those animals may be contributing to your child's occasional misery, and that continually being exposed to those allergens may make a mild case of allergies worse.

15 SMART SOLUTION
Establish a smoke-free house.

Children who live in households with smokers are at a greater risk of developing respiratory disease. Children have a lifetime for the harmful products contained in tobacco smoke to wreak havoc on their bodies. But tobacco smoke isn't the only smoke in a home that can cause problems.

☆☆☆
Very
Important

△△
Moderately
Easy

Wood-burning stoves and fireplaces can give off all kinds of toxic materials, including benzene, formaldehyde, and carbon monoxide. Children who are exposed to wood smoke are more likely to have chronic cough, wheezing, and asthma attacks than other children. These children may also be at greater risk for lung cancer because the tars and tiny particles produced in wood smoke are similar to those produced in tobacco smoke.

You can enjoy your wood-burning stove or fireplace, though, without endangering the health your child. First, make sure your wood-burning stove or fireplace has an adequate draft. The smoke should go up the chimney, not into your room. Second, if you have a wood-burning stove, have the catalytic converter and the chimney checked and cleaned once a year to make sure they're working as efficiently as possible. (You also might want to visit the Environmental Protection Agency's Web site at www.epa.gov for regulatory information on wood-burning stoves.)

Fumes from stoves and furnaces can give off carbon monoxide. This odorless, colorless gas may not be detected before it reaches lethal levels, which is why it's extremely dangerous. Your best defense against potential problems with carbon monoxide fumes from gas stoves, wood stoves, and hot-water heaters is to have them checked annually for proper combustion and venting. Old chimneys can develop leaks, and chimney flues can become clogged, too, allowing life-threatening carbon monoxide to seep into your house. So it's also important to have your chimney cleaned and checked annually. And it's well worth it to invest in a carbon-monoxide detector with a digital readout that will alert you to dangerous levels of this gas. A digital readout enables you to determine the actual level of carbon monoxide in the room and will help you determine whether you have a severely malfunctioning unit or one that produces borderline levels of carbon monoxide. (You might want to check out *Consumer Reports* for information about specific models and performance; see "Recommended Reading" on page 144.)

BREAKING THE HABIT

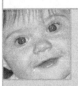 IF YOU'RE a parent who smokes, we strongly encourage you to stop smoking. We know it's hard to do. Members of our families are ex-smokers, and we experienced first-hand with them the difficulties of stopping. But we all agree it's really worth the effort. And now is a great time to stop smoking, as you have years ahead of you to enjoy free breathing.

Many different strategies are available to help you stop—from nicotine gum and hypnotism to antidepressant medication and nicotine patches. Talk to your family doctor or call your local chapter of the American Lung Association to find out about the right way for you. If you stop, you'll be rewarded with more stamina—and maybe even a better sex life (did you know smoking is linked to impotence?). You'll also greatly increase your chance of being around to enjoy a hike in the woods with your children and grandchildren in the years to come.

Gas stoves produce nitrogen dioxide and other respiratory irritants. Stoves with gas pilot lights are particularly troublesome since they produce these gases day and night. If you have a gas stove, frequently ventilate your house to help reduce these irritants. And the next time you buy a gas stove, you may wish to choose one without a pilot light. Many gas stoves now have an electronic ignition that produces a spark when you turn on the burner. The spark, in turn, lights the burner.

Oil-burning furnaces produce fumes that can be toxic if you don't have adequate ventilation in your home. Spilled or leaking fuel oil can introduce toxic chemicals into the air; it can also find its way into well water when there are wells in the vicinity of the spill. Scrupulous maintenance of your oil burner, annual checkups on efficiency and ventilation, and regular cleanings for the chimney and filters are the best ways to prevent problems with your oil furnace.

Gasoline and kerosene home heaters produce toxic substances—including soot, which can cause cancer, and carbon monoxide, which can cause death by asphyxiation. Worst of all is that gasoline and kerosene heaters can accidentally tip over, spill burning fuel, and cause terrible burns. The best defense against these problems is to avoid using these heaters. If you currently have a gasoline or kerosene heater, replace it with an electric heater, preferably one that doesn't get hot to the touch.

16 SMART SOLUTION
Air out your house.

Is the air in your house polluted? Before you say no, consider that in most areas, indoor air has more pollutants than outdoor air. If you have any of these in your home, you may have indoor air pollution.

☆ **Good Idea**

△ **Easy**

- ☐ Rugs and carpets
- ☐ Curtains
- ☐ Cleaning products
- ☐ Nail polish remover
- ☐ Hair spray
- ☐ Shoe polish
- ☐ Potpourri

- ☐ Furniture
- ☐ Dog and cat hair
- ☐ Cockroach droppings
- ☐ Secondhand tobacco smoke
- ☐ Furnaces
- ☐ Gas stoves
- ☐ Wood-burning stoves and fireplaces

In other words, almost all homes have some sources of indoor air pollution. To keep air pollutants from building up, take the simple step of airing out your house once a week.

To air out your house, choose a bright, clear day, open your windows, and let the air blow through your house. On cold winter days, you might even consider turning off your heat and opening up your whole house for an hour or so. What you lose in energy efficiency is offset by what you gain in restoring humidity and fresh, clean air to your house.

Of course, sometimes the outdoor air quality won't be very good. Particular pollens in the air, for example, cause

INDUSTRIAL POLLUTANTS

TOXIC EMISSIONS (toxic pollutants that industries emit into the air) can produce an unhealthy chemical soup. So if you live near an industry that emits pollutants into the air, find out what chemicals are emitted and where the wind patterns take them. Under the Superfund Reauthorization Act, the Environmental Protection Agency (EPA) and local governments must maintain registries of industrial chemical releases. Contact your local or state health department to learn about permitted emissions in your area. Or log on to www.scorecard.org, a Web site maintained by Environmental Defense that provides toxic emission data. At this site, you can actually find out the type and amount of pollution that exists, as well as where it's coming from, in the area of the country where you live.

PROBLEM POLLENS

 THE FOLLOWING list includes plants that produce allergy-triggering pollens. If your child is allergic to certain pollens, you might want to consider investing in an electric air cleaner with a HEPA (high-efficiency particulate air) filter to remove pollen from the air indoors. If you can keep only one room pollen-free, your child's bedroom is a good choice.

Weeds	Grasses	Trees
English plantain	Bermudagrass	Ash
Lamb's-quarters	Johnsongrass	Box elder
Ragweed	Kentucky bluegrass	Elm
Redroot pigweed	Orchardgrass	Hickory
Sagebrush	Redtop	Mountain cedar
Tumbleweed	Sweet vernal	Oak
	Timothy	Pecan

allergies. The weather report on your local news channel or the national Weather Channel are often good sources to turn to find out about the pollen count in your area.

Ozone levels and toxic emissions are two other sources of outdoor air pollution to consider before opening up your house. Ozone is a respiratory irritant formed when sunlight acts on automobile exhaust fumes and industrial pollution. In some parts of the country, "ozone alerts" are issued by state and federal agencies and are common during the hot, humid days of summer. Listen for these alerts, and don't air out your house when ozone levels are high.

17 SMART SOLUTION
Clean up the air indoors.

As we just mentioned in Smart Solution 16, airing out your house is a good way to keep air pollutants from building up inside your home. Another thing you can do to keep the air in your house from becoming a chemical soup is to choose and use household products (such as cleaning supplies and paint removers) wisely.

Important

Moderately
Easy

The following is a list of household products that contain respiratory irritants and toxic chemicals, as well as how you can minimize the dangers from them.

Extremely Toxic

Drain cleaners. Your best bet when it comes to drain cleaners is to avoid using them. Most drain cleaners contain lye (sodium hydroxide), which can cause severe burns—and can be life threatening if a child drinks it. Instead, try a nontoxic method of fixing the problem. Pour 1 cup of baking soda and 1 cup of vinegar down the drain. Follow the baking soda and vinegar with boiling water to help break the clog. If your sink is draining slowly, you can try to take apart the drain mechanism and remove the clog by hand.

Oven cleaners. Lye is also the active ingredient in many oven cleaners. Because lye is so dangerous, it's best to avoid lye-based oven cleaners, especially those in aerosol cans. While aerosols assure that the material is evenly dispersed in your oven, they also coat your hair, skin, and lungs with fine droplets. As an alternative to using lye-based oven cleaners, warm the oven, then moisten the dirty parts with water, sprinkle them with baking soda, wait a few minutes, then scrub with steel wool until clean. Or, try Arm & Hammer Oven Cleaner, which is nontoxic.

If you feel you have to use a lye-based cleaner, avoid products that need to be used on a warm or hot oven: The combination will produce additional respiratory irritants. Also choose a "paint-on" type of lye that's impregnated in a steel wool base (which at least assures that you're not inhaling the lye to the same extent that you would with the other types of lye products).

Petroleum-based polyurethane floor and furniture finishes. These products contain several highly toxic substances, including toluene di-isocyanate (TDI). When inhaled, TDI can cause airway sensitivity, and reexposure to TDI can cause chemically induced asthma. So choose

---

SMART SHOPPING

 IF YOU absolutely need to use a lye-based product to clean your drains or oven, purchase it right before you're going to use it, in the smallest amount necessary. Always keep it in a locked cabinet, out of reach of children. Lye can severely burn a child's esophagus and lungs if ingested and can be life-threatening. Use the product immediately (make sure the room is well ventilated when you do use it), and discard anything that's left over promptly and safely.

water-based polyurethane floor and furniture finishes, which are safer and less toxic. And always make sure your house is well ventilated when you're applying polyurethane, then air out the house for a few days afterward.

Paint removers. Most paint removers can be very dangerous. Products containing methylene chloride, for example, are highly toxic and can cause severe blood and liver problems when their fumes are inhaled. If you need to use paint remover, choose products without methylene chloride, such as 3M Safest Stripper. Keep in mind that you still need adequate ventilation with these products—and you need to follow the product label instructions.

Moderately Toxic

Mildew removers. Some mildew removers contain sodium metabisulfite, a chemical that produces an extremely potent respiratory irritant, sulfur dioxide. This irritant can trigger severe respiratory distress in sensitive people. Look for mildew removers that contain chlorine bleach, as these will do the job without triggering respiratory attacks. Or make a dilute solution of chlorine bleach and water (¼ cup bleach per gallon of water) to clean mildew. Always make sure to use these solutions in a room with good ventilation.

Craft (airplane) glue. Most of the glues used to put together models contain substances that can be hazardous to kids. Solvents in some craft glues are neurotoxins, which can damage a child's developing brain and nervous system and can even be lethal. In fact, each year children are brought to the hospital with neurotoxicity related to glue sniffing (when kids intentionally sniff glue to get high).

Even if your child is using the glue as it was meant to be used—for building a model—she can still experience toxic effects from the glue such as dizziness or blurred vision, depending on the size of the room she's working in, how well it's ventilated, and how much glue she's using. Our advice is to use nontoxic alternatives, such as wood or white glue, for these projects. If those glues won't work, use the smallest amount of craft glue necessary in a well-ventilated room. Air out the room frequently, and have your child leave the room regularly so she's not continually being exposed to the glue's fumes.

POTPOURRI'S PLEASANT ODOR CAN ALSO BE A RESPIRATORY IRRITANT TO BABIES AND TODDLERS, AND IT CAN COLLECT DUST AS WELL. IT'S BETTER TO AVOID IT ALTOGETHER.

Minor Irritants

Fingernail polish remover. Many of these products contain acetone, a toxic solvent that vaporizes readily. Try the nonacetone products, which generally contain solvents that don't vaporize as easily (look for "acetone-free" labels on the bottles). If you or your child must use an acetone product, do so in a well-ventilated room. And never let your child spend hours in a fingernail salon—where larger quantities of acetone and other solvents are used—while you're having your nails done.

Hair spray. This beauty product can contain lacquers and other ingredients that may be respiratory irritants to children. And using hair spray in a small, confined space such as your bathroom can build up the levels of irritants rapidly, especially if you're using an aerosol can. So choose products with nonaerosol cans, and use them in a well-ventilated area.

Newly painted walls. Fresh paint emits solvents as it dries. Ventilate your house well for several days to a few weeks after painting to minimize the buildup of chemicals. Also, choose water-based paints, which generally have fewer toxic solvents than oil-based paints.

New furniture and rugs. New furniture and rugs can contain formaldehyde and other chemical solvents, which is what accounts for that "new" smell. Formaldehyde, however, is a potent carcinogen and respiratory toxin. So ventilate your house well every day for several days to several weeks after buying new furniture or rugs to minimize the buildup of formaldehyde and other chemicals from these products. Washing or airing out cotton or synthetic rugs until the "new" smell disappears is also a good idea.

18 SMART SOLUTION
Eliminate roaches safely.

Roaches can show up in homes in all parts of the country (no matter how clean your house is), although they're most likely to appear in urban or apartment housing, where many dwelling units occupy a small area. And one of the bad things about these nasty critters is that recent studies show roach droppings can trigger allergies and asthma in kids.

☆☆
Important

△△
Moderately
Easy

If you have roaches, though, don't reach for a can of pesticide to wipe them out because pesticides are toxic to the brain and nervous system. And in some people, asthma attacks follow the use of certain types of pesticides. Although the relationship between children, pesticides, and asthma still hasn't been nailed down, your best bet is to walk on the safe side and avoid using chemical pesticides. (See Smart Solutions 30 32 for more information on the hazards of using pesticides.)

To get rid of roaches in a safe, nontoxic way, try some or all of the following tactics.

Set out glue traps. Place these traps wherever you see roaches, and remove and replace them as they do their job.

Sprinkle boric acid. Wash down the kitchen cabinet shelves and replace the shelf liner with nonsticky paper, then sprinkle boric acid underneath the paper. Do not use boric acid on shelves that your kids or pets can reach—or else keep those cabinets locked. Also sprinkle boric acid in hard-to-reach places where roaches hang out, such as behind the refrigerator and stove.

Enforce a "no food in the bedroom" rule. Food attracts roaches, so confine the cookie and pizza crumbs to the kitchen and dining areas, where you can easily sweep them up. Keeping the children's rooms off-limits for food will minimize the likelihood that roaches will settle there and trigger allergies while the children sleep.

Dry the kitchen before bedtime. Roaches like water sources and consider damp sponges and wet dishes left in the sink as an open invitation to stop by. So dry those dishes and put those wet sponges in a plastic bag. Before storing a sponge in a plastic bag overnight, make sure you wash it thoroughly in hot, soapy water. Wash it again in the morning to minimize any buildup of germs. You can also stick your sponge in the dishwasher and wash it along with your dishes to keep it clean and fresh.

Clean up dark corners. Grease and crumbs that accumulate in hard-to-reach places can support entire families of roaches. So periodically clean up food residue from under the refrigerator, behind the stove, and in other out-of-the-way nooks and crannies in your kitchen.

Seal cracks and crevices. Cracks and crevices in the walls, floors, and corners where the walls and floor meet can serve as secret hideaways for roaches and enable them to move from room to room without you noticing them. You can fill small cracks with caulking compound similar to what you use to seal the seam between the tile and your bathtub. Fill larger cracks with wood shim and then caulk. Choose a nontoxic caulk meant for indoor use.

10 Practical Tips for Preventing Lead Poisoning

IN THIS day and age, do you really still need to worry about lead poisoning? Absolutely. Lead is a toxic substance that can damage the kidneys, heart, and gastrointestinal system and can lead to brain damage. At high levels, lead poisoning can cause seizures. Granted, severe cases of lead poisoning have become less common as medical treatment and efforts at prevention have become more sophisticated. However, you still need to be concerned because even low levels of lead can damage the developing brain and nervous system of a child.

Studies have shown that children with even small amounts of lead in their blood have more difficulty learning and have lower intelligence quotients (IQ) than children without lead in their blood. For every 10 ug/dl (micrograms per deciliter) of lead in the blood, a child's IQ may drop 2 to 4 points.

You may not think that losing 2 to 4 IQ points is significant—but losing even just a few means that your child may not reach his full potential. If your child has marginal intelligence, lead poisoning could make the difference between his ability to function as a full member of society and being a child whose full potential may not be reached because of lead poisoning. Lead poisoning could be equally as devastating if your child is gifted, perhaps robbing our society of an Einstein or a Mozart.

In addition to affecting intelligence, lead poisoning may also cause behavioral problems, including a shortened attention span. Researchers have shown that young men (under 18 years old) jailed for juvenile delinquency have higher levels of lead in their bodies than other young men from the same neighborhoods who have no criminal record.

The effects of lead poisoning (which are permanent) can occur silently and may often cause no symptoms. The good news, though, is that it is possible to prevent your child from being exposed to lead—and it's not hard to do. Here are some practical ways to get started.

19 SMART SOLUTION
Be your own Sherlock Holmes.

The first step in preventing your child from being exposed to lead is to be a household detective. Check for peeling and chipping paint—the number-one cause of lead poisoning in children—inside and outside your house. The Children's Health Environmental Coalition has developed an excellent workbook, *The Household Detective,* that you may want to use as you do your household investigation. See "Resources" on page 145 for their contact information.

☆☆☆
Very
Important

△
Easy

If your house was built before 1970, it probably has lead paint in it—the federal government didn't ban the use of lead paint in houses until a few years later. When lead paint flakes, it creates lead dust and chips that fall on the floor and collect in window wells and on windowsills, floor moldings, and other flat places in your house. Young children, especially infants and children younger than 6 years, are at a health risk from this lead paint and dust.

Lead gets into the bodies of children in a variety of ways. Kids can ingest the dust after putting toys—or even their hands—that have lead dust on them in their mouths. (And as you well know, infants and toddlers put *everything* in their mouths.) When toddlers are tall enough to look out the window, they often use the windowsill as a teething ring.

And not only is it pretty easy for kids to get lead paint into their mouths, it's also tasty to them because it's sweet. In fact, children can actually develop a craving for lead paint (this is called "pica"). Some kids like the taste of lead paint so much that they become quite persistent in finding and eating paint chips.

The easiest thing you can do to help protect your children from exposure to lead paint is to make sure you don't have any in your home. Here are a list of places where you'd commonly find chipping and peeling paint. Thoroughly check out each area and note what you find—and then have those areas tested for lead.

Window wells. The window well is the part of the window that is exposed at the bottom when you open it. So open the window and take a peek. Does the paint have a cracked (crazed) surface that looks like alligator skin? Are there chips of paint visible? Do there seem to be many layers of paint in the well? If so, this area may contain lead paint.

Window and door frames. Is there flaking, peeling, or chipping paint where friction occurs? Is there visible chipping, flaking, or cracking (crazing)? Is there paint dust on the floor or wallboard?

Plaster walls. Pay particular attention to areas under the windows and in places where leaks or moisture may have caused some damage to the surface of the paint. Are chips, flakes, or dust apparent?

Stairs, banisters, old cast-iron radiators, and chair rails. Again, look for signs of flaking, peeling, and chipping paint. Also check out other wooden surfaces in your home that are subject to wear and tear.

The outside of your house. Lead paint may likely have been used on the trim or the siding of the house. Are these areas in good condition? Check the garage and garden storage

A LESSON IN LEAD

HOW DO we know that lead levels affect intelligence? In 1976, Herbert Needleman, M.D., then a researcher at Harvard Medical School, began an innovative longitudinal study of first- and second-grade public school students in Somerville and Chelsea, Massachusetts. About 2,500 children from 29 schools volunteered to bring in their baby teeth when they fell out. (Lead levels in teeth and bones are indicative of lead exposure.) Researchers measured the lead levels in their teeth and compared each child's school progress and teacher ratings to the level of exposure to lead.

Then, in 1977 and 1978, the researchers followed up on the same children and administered psychological tests. They found that higher lead levels in baby teeth were associated with decreased IQ, poorer attention span, and impaired language function. In 1988, the researchers contacted half of the original sample of children and found that those who had high lead levels in their baby teeth were seven times as likely to fail to graduate from high school and six times as likely to have a reading disability than those children without high levels of lead.

LEAD-TESTING CAUTIONS

HAVING PAINT chips tested by a laboratory or by using lead-detecting crayons (usually sold in hardware stores) are two ways to test for lead paint. But each of these methods has significant drawbacks. If you decide to send a paint chip to a laboratory for lead testing, be sure that the laboratory is certified for lead paint testing by your state or local government or by the EPA (Environmental Protection Agency). Then keep in mind that the paint chip you send is only one sample of what exists in your house. It may not be representative of the paint used in every room. Even if it comes back negative, that shows only that there is no lead paint in that chip. That doesn't mean you don't have lead paint elsewhere in your home.

The lead-detecting crayons also suffer from a problem: If layers of latex paint have been painted over old lead paint, the crayon may not be able to detect the underlying lead. Later, if the latex paint chips and peels, you may be exposing your child to lead paint that exists under the layers of latex paint.

Ultimately, the best way to have your paint tested for lead is through XRF detection. (See below.)

area as well as fences and porch railings. Also, take a look at the sandbox or play area—is it so close to the house that it might be contaminated by peeling or chipping paint?

If you find any chipping or peeling paint, have it tested to find out whether it's lead-based. If you don't own your own home, let your landlord know if you've seen signs of peeling or chipping paint, and ask him for evidence that the home or apartment has been tested for lead. If it hasn't been tested, ask to have it done.

The most definitive way to find out if you have lead in your house is by having your walls and trim examined through x-ray fluorescence (XRF), especially those areas where you suspect you may have a problem. Contact your local or state health department for names of certified lead paint abatement (removal) professionals in your area who are qualified to do a household paint inspection with an XRF detector. Using this method is the only way of being sure your house is safe. Even if the tests show there is no lead in your house, the cost is well worth the peace of mind you'll have knowing that your children are safe from lead poisoning.

20 SMART SOLUTION
Call in a professional.

When dealing with a potential lead paint problem, you want the best information available. A certified lead inspector who's been trained in lead paint assessment and abatement is the best person to turn to. Some states require that workers who perform lead paint abatement be certified (see "States with Certification" on page 36 for states that currently mandate this certification), while other states haven't passed laws requiring certification for lead paint abatement workers.

☆☆☆
Very Important

△
Easy

If you live in a state without mandatory certification, use a contractor who has passed certification courses that meet the EPA training guidelines—and ask to see documentation of his certification. Visit www.leadlisting.org for a list of lead-trained renovators in your region. When in doubt, call your state or local health department for information.

21 SMART SOLUTION
Get rid of lead paint the right way.

The best way to remove lead paint is to have it done by a certified lead abatement contractor. (See Smart Solution [19]) But if you decide to remove lead paint yourself, it's important to do it right. Many families have developed lead poisoning when they attempted to do household renovations themselves. Here's a typical story of how that happens.

☆☆☆
Very Important

△△△
Difficult

A young family moves into a beautiful old house that needs a lot of work. Paint is peeling and flaking on both the inside and outside of the house. The doors and woodwork are chipped, and the floor in the baby's room is painted an awful color.

So the family begins renovations. Over the next week, they sand the outside trim with an electric sander, although no one realizes the dust is blowing into the house through the open windows. Once they notice all the dust inside, out comes the vacuum cleaner to suck it up.

They also rent a floor sander to get rid of the paint on the baby's room floor. The sander has a vacuum bag attachment that's supposed to keep the dust down. When the floor is finished, though, a fine layer of powdery dust covers everything in the house—including the dinner dishes. Then, they use a heat gun to remove the chipping paint from the woodwork.

STATES WITH CERTIFICATION

HERE'S A list of states that mandate certification for lead paint abatement inspectors.

	Iowa	New	Utah
	Kentucky	Hampshire	Virginia
Alabama	Kansas	New Jersey	Vermont
Arkansas	Louisiana	North	Washington,
California	Massachusetts	Carolina	D.C.
Colorado	Maryland	Ohio	West Virginia
Connecticut	Maine	Oklahoma	Wisconsin
Delaware	Michigan	Oregon	
Georgia	Minnesota	Pennsylvania	
Illinois	Mississippi	Rhode Island	
Indiana	Missouri	Texas	

That night after using the heat gun, all the family members are a bit queasy and have a nasty headache. The next day, the dog starts acting ill. He's so sick, in fact, that they stop working on the house to take him to the vet, where the vet suggests the dog has lead poisoning.

A hasty trip to their family physician follows. Tests confirm the baby has lead poisoning, too, and is going to need to be hospitalized for chelation therapy. (Chelation involves giving a person oral or intravenous medication to speed the elimination of lead from his body. The lead in the body becomes bound or "chelated" to the medication and is excreted along with the medication in the person's urine.) The doctor says the baby will probably be fine, but that it's too soon to tell whether she'll have any lasting effects from the lead poisoning.

What Went Wrong?

Sanding lead paint causes lead dust to spread everywhere—in this case, it fell throughout the house, into the dirt outside, and into the sandbox. Using an ordinary vacuum to suck up the dust just spread the lead even further—into the curtains, furniture, clothes, and cupboards, and onto the countertops (where it ended up in the sugar bowl and on the plate of cookies). Using the heat gun to remove the paint from the window trim wasn't a good idea either; the heat gun actually vaporized the lead. And the surest way to get lead poisoning is to inhale lead fumes.

Obviously, if you have home remodeling to do, you don't want to end up like the family in this example. Here are some tips that may help you avoid their fate.

- Assume any paint applied before 1976 is lead paint.

- Learn how to properly and safely remove the paint before starting. You can get more information from the National Lead Information Center at 1-800-LEAD-FYI. Also check out *Reducing Lead Hazards When Remodeling Your Home,* published by the EPA (see "Resources" on page 145), or call your local or state health department for helpful information. Or visit the Web site of the Alliance to End Childhood Lead Poisoning at www.aeclp.org.

- Wear approved respiratory protection and appropriate clothing, and be sure to wash it separately from your other dirty laundry. *Reducing Lead Hazards When Remodeling Your Home* lists specific respiratory protection and clothing needed to help you avoid exposure to lead dust.

- Never sand lead paint. Sanding creates lead dust that can spread throughout your house.

- Never use a heat gun to remove lead paint because the heat will vaporize the lead and disperse it into the air.

22 SMART SOLUTION
Temporarily relocate children and pregnant women during lead paint removal.

Children and pregnant women should live with relatives or friends when you or a professional are doing lead paint abatement work in your home. They shouldn't return until all the debris and dust has been thoroughly cleaned up and the house is safe from lead hazards. Because a child's nervous system is still developing, direct exposure leaves him at high risk for lead poisoning. And a pregnant woman can experience miscarriage, stillbirth, premature delivery, or premature rupture of membranes due to lead poisoning at high lead levels—or have a baby whose developing brain has been damaged by the lead.

☆☆☆
Very
Important

Difficult

23 SMART SOLUTION
Make sure your drinking water is lead-free.

Although the majority of lead poisoning in children is caused by lead paint, other sources of lead can contribute to lead poisoning, including the water your child drinks.

☆
Good
Idea

That's right—you might even have lead in your water. Here's how it gets there.

△
Easy

Some older communities have lead pipes delivering their municipal water supplies. Over the years, the pipes become coated on the inside with a "biofilm," a layer of organic material that acts to keep the lead from coming in direct contact with the water. In places where the municipal water is acidic, however, the acid eats away at the biofilm, causing the lead to leach from the pipes into the water.

Most lead in drinking water, though, comes from a home's plumbing. In the early and mid-1900s, lead pipes were commonly used for household plumbing. So if you have an old house and the plumbing has never been updated, you may have a lead problem in your water.

Take a few minutes to check out your pipes. Lead pipes are generally a dull gray, and the metal is somewhat soft. Other materials used for household plumbing include cast-iron and copper. Cast-iron pipes are usually black and hard; if they're galvanized, they may appear gray but aren't soft. Copper piping is the typical copper color. Even if you have copper piping, however, you might still have lead in your water because there may have been lead in the solder used to join the pipes together. Lead solder has been banned only since 1986.

If you have lead or copper pipes in your home, you'll want to know for certain if they're leaching lead into your water. If you are served by municipal water, you should receive notification from your city's water supplier if you have lead in your water: In 1991 the Environmental Protection Agency put into effect its "Lead and Copper Rule," which requires water suppliers to notify their customers if lead or copper levels in their water exceed standards set by the federal government. In addition, all water companies are required to send out an annual report on contaminants to their customers.

If you have well water, you should have your water tested for lead content at a certified laboratory. Contact your local or state health department for certified laboratories near you.

Having lead in your water doesn't necessarily mean you need to replace the plumbing in your home. In most cases, the easiest way to eliminate any lead in your drinking or cooking water before drinking it or using it for cooking is to run the cold water for 30 seconds or so after it has sat in the pipes for hours at a time—such as after work or school, or first thing in the morning. Because water from a municipal supplier is generally lead free, running the water before using it lets you access lead-free water from the water mains rather than the water that has leached lead from your house-hold plumbing while sitting in the pipes. And always use *cold* water to drink, cook, and make baby formula—hot water can leach more lead from the household plumbing. (If you're on a well, you should still run the water for 30 sec-onds after it's been sitting around for a while to be safe.)

24 SMART SOLUTION
Have your child's blood tested for lead.

Lead poisoning has been recognized since antiquity. In fact, the fall of Rome may have been caused by lead poi-soning, as lead aqueducts carried drinking water throughout the city and lead was used as a sweetener for wine.

☆☆
Important

△
Easy

What's new about lead poisoning is just now being dis-covered during this century. Sophisticated technology allows us to measure and track minute quantities of lead in the body. We can now see what lead is doing to the very cells and molecules that make up our brain and nervous system. And what we're learning is alarming.

Over the course of the past few decades, the Centers for Disease Control and Prevention (CDC) has continued to lower the acceptable blood levels of lead in children. What was once considered safe is now known to be dangerous. Over a dozen studies conducted by different researchers during the 1980s and 1990s show measurable adverse health effects at blood lead levels as low as 10 ug/dl, a level once considered safe, but now labeled as dangerous by the CDC.

The average blood lead level of most people in the United States, including most children between 1 and 5 years of age, is 2.8 ug/dl. A generation ago, the average blood lead for Americans of all ages was between 18 and 20 ug/dl, when leaded gasoline was in general use. However, today nearly 1 million children in the United States still have blood lead levels greater than 10 ug/dl.

The only way to be sure your child doesn't have lead poi-soning is to have her receive a blood test for lead annually until age 6. This lead test is especially important for children between the ages of 1 and 3 who live in or visit homes built before 1970 because they are at highest risk for lead poisoning. (Your doctor can perform a simple fingerstick in his office and have an accurate result in 2 minutes.)

25 SMART SOLUTION
Keep things clean.

If you have lead paint in your house, mop weekly with a mild detergent solution from the floor up the walls to the height of your child plus 1 foot. Many grocery stores and home centers carry nontoxic soaps that you can dilute to make just such a mild cleaning solution. Cleaning up will help get rid of the lead dust before it gets into your child.

Important

Easy

Use paper towels to wipe down windowsills, window wells, baseboards, floor and door moldings, wall trims, and other flat places. Seeing things from your child's point of view will also help you figure out which nooks and crannies to clean. Sit on the floor and move around the room, removing dust from every place your child can reach. Put the used paper towels in a secure trash container so they don't dry out and redistribute the lead dust around the house.

In addition to washing your floors and other surfaces weekly, regularly wash your child's toys and pacifiers. Wash your child's hands frequently as well, especially before he sits down for a meal or snack.

26 SMART SOLUTION
Make sure your child's toys are lead-free.

During the past several years, lead has been found in a number of toys. Recalls or product warnings due to lead content have included:

- Crayons made in China

- China tea sets for dollhouses

- Painted toys imported from Mexico and China

- Lead figurines used in games for children and teens

Before purchasing toys, make sure they are lead-free—that is, purchase toys made in this country, where lead testing is done. If you purchase toys from other countries, do so with caution, as not all countries test their products for lead.

27 SMART SOLUTION
Check out your dinnerware.

Pottery made in the United States is required to pass inspections that assure that it's lead-free. Pottery from other countries, however, may contain lead. And when the glazing is imperfect, lead can leach from the pottery into your food.

The worst type of problem with improperly glazed pottery occurs when you store an acidic liquid, such as orange juice, in the pottery. The acid in the orange juice can dissolve the lead. So, to be on the safe side, don't use lead pottery for storing any acidic liquid.

Highly glazed china and coffee cups may also contain lead. The brighter the color, the higher your level of suspicion should be. The best and brightest colors seem to be lead based.

Older pots and pans with chipped enamel can be a source of lead poisoning, too, because the metal under the enamel may contain lead. Cooking foods—especially acidic foods like tomato sauce—in these pans can cause the lead to leach from the pan into your food. Pots and pans made today in the United States should be lead-free.

☆ Good Idea

△ Easy

28 SMART SOLUTION
Keep the sandbox away from the house.

If you have lead paint on the outside of your house, make sure the sandbox is at least 5 feet away from the side of the house. You don't want lead paint to flake off and land in your child's sandbox. Also, teach your kids not to play in the dirt near the house, and plant shrubs or groundcover to keep the dirt from becoming dusty. The last thing you want is for your kids to inhale dust particles with lead in them.

☆ Good Idea

△ Easy

CHOOSE LEAD-FREE CANDLES

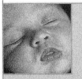 YOU MIGHT like to add sparkle to your home with lighted candles, particularly on special occasions. However, some candles on the market (mostly imported ones) contain lead in their wicks. The problem is that a candle with a leaded wick can produce lead fumes as it burns, causing a serious hazard if the fumes are inhaled. Although the Consumer Product Safety Commission voted to ban candles with lead in their wicks in 2001, you should still make sure that any candles you buy are certified to be lead-free.

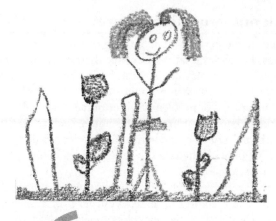

6 Cautions about Pesticides and Herbicides

WHEN YOU spray pesticides to kill garden or household critters, douse your lawn with chemical herbicides, or spray your dog for fleas, you're also exposing your kids (and yourself) to these toxins. Think about it: These concoctions are designed to *kill* insects and weeds. Even if you use them as directed, they still have the potential to cause a wide range of health problems in people because of their toxicity. Some alarming thoughts:

No one guarantees the safety of pesticides. Just because a product is registered with the Environmental Protection Agency (EPA) doesn't mean it's safe. Registration of a pesticide by the EPA isn't a human health risk assessment. It's a process that balances the benefits of the pesticide with the potential risks of the product. All pesticides are dangerous, although not to the same degree.

Pesticides have been traditionally treated as "innocent until proven guilty" by regulatory authorities. A generation ago, pesticides were considered to be relatively safe and effective chemicals that produced significant benefits to society. Deadly diseases spread by insects, such as malaria and yellow fever, were brought under control through the use of pesticides. Pesticides also greatly increased the production of food and farm products. Their health effects were not well understood, so at that time they were allowed to become part of our daily lives without being subject to adequate testing.

Many older pesticides have not been thoroughly tested by today's standards. These pesticides are still commonly used even though complete testing of these older pesticides will take at least another 10 years.

Most pesticides in use today have not been tested for their health effects on children. This is a major problem. Recent scientific studies involving laboratory animals show that many pesticides damage the developing brain and nervous system. This is a significant concern when it comes to kids because they're much more vulnerable than adults to chemicals that interfere with their rapidly developing brains and nervous systems. Behavioral problems and deficits in the ability to learn are only a few of the problems that can result from interference with the normal development of a child's brain and nervous system.

Certain types of pesticides mimic hormones. Scientists have discovered that some pesticides have the ability to mimic or compete with hormones (the chemicals in our body that trigger development and functioning). These substances may interfere with normal body development and functioning, especially of the reproductive system and the thyroid. Our body requires only minuscule amounts of these various hormones to produce the desired effects—so if we receive too many in the form of pesticides, they may wreak havoc with our bodies. This is especially true if exposure takes place during critical windows of vulnerability early in a child's development.

Many herbicides are known, probable, or suspected carcinogens (cancer-causing chemicals). Phenoxy herbicides, for example, are members of the same chemical family as the notorious Agent Orange used widely in the Vietnam War. These herbicides can contain dioxin, a cancer-causing chemical. Studies show that one type of cancer—non-Hodgkin's lymphoma—is more common in farmers and in workers in factories that make herbicides that contain phenoxy. Herbicides with phenoxy in them (2,4-D, for example) are available in most garden, home, and hardware stores. Is that what your want on your lawn, where your children play and your pets romp?

Our point is that you do have lots of nontoxic options when it comes to eliminating bugs and weeds, so why needlessly expose your children to chemicals that may harm their health? Here are some alternatives.

29 SMART SOLUTION
Keep pests under control.

You might think that zapping insects with a can of bug spray is the best way to eliminate less-than-desirable creepy-crawlies. And while pesticides are obviously designed to kill bugs, they do so only to an extent. They wipe out the weaker bugs, but the stronger ones tend to survive and multiply—what's known as "survival of the fittest." What ends up happening is that the pests develop a resistance to the pesticide, so it loses its effectiveness.

☆☆
Important

△△
Moderately Easy

Pesticides also don't distinguish between good and bad bugs—so when you're out spraying your vegetable or flower garden, you're killing off all the butterflies, bees, beetles, and other helpful insects that are necessary for pollination and that also prey on bad bugs. And while you're dousing bugs with pesticides, you're exposing your children to toxic chemicals that can harm their health.

You can beat bad bugs both in and outside your home, though, with an approach called Integrated Pest Management (IPM). (See Smart Solution 85) Instead of fighting pests with chemicals, IPM starts with the premise that pests need to be kept under control, not eliminated as a species. IPM calls for the use of the least-toxic substances available and the smallest quantities needed to do the job. In IPM, chemical pesticides are the weapon of last resort, not the first line of defense.

An easy way to keep pests under control in your home using IPM is to take away their food and water. Wipe down your kitchen sink and counters each evening so that the creepy-crawlies will have nothing to drink. Make sure you wipe up all the crumbs on counters, as well as sweep up any crumbs that are on the kitchen floor. Every month or two, pull your refrigerator out from the wall, and clean up any food residues under it. Use wood shims or caulk to seal off any cracks and crevices in your kitchen walls or in the corners between walls and floors so the pests will have nowhere to run and hide. If, after those efforts, you still have a pest problem, choose the least-toxic options: Combat brand bait or gel, or boric acid, but not chemical strips or sprays.

For more detailed information on IPM, see "Resources" on page 145 or call your local cooperative extension office—you'll find their number in your phone book.

30
Avoid organophosphates.

Organophosphates are a class of pesticides that are extremely toxic; they can even be life-threatening if accidental exposure occurs. Pesticide poisonings from organophosphates can result if the pesticide comes in contact with your skin, you breathe the vapors, or you ingest the material. Symptoms include blurred vision, abdominal pain, increased salivation, sweating, irritability, nausea, vomiting, muscle spasms, mental confusion, and seizures.

☆☆☆
Very
Important

△
Easy

Probably the most well-known organophosphate is chlorpyrifos, which is the active ingredient in many pesticides, including Dursban and Lorsban. Although the EPA has sharply reduced the use of chlorpyrifos because of concerns about children's health, it's still available in products on hardware, home center, and garden store shelves. Chlorpyrifos is used to kill fleas, bees, wasps, hornets, termites, and roaches. This

BEWARE OF THESE POISONS

CHLORPYRIFOS ISN'T the only organophosphate on the market. Others to avoid include:

Malathion. This pesticide is found in products designed to eliminate household pests, flies, and mosquitoes. Although it's one of the less-toxic organophosphates, you should still avoid using it. Many nontoxic techniques, such as a strong spray of water, work just fine for ridding houseplants of pest insects like aphids.

Diazinon. This organophosphate is a pesticide that's sold widely in lawn, garden, and hardware stores. Although diazinon is being phased out by the EPA, it will be available in many stores until 2004. And, in fact, its sales are expected to increase as the new federal restrictions on chlorpyrifos come into force. Diazinon hasn't been tested as rigorously as chlorpyrifos, but it may well pose many of the same risks to the developing brain and nervous system of a child.

Methyl parathion. This highly toxic organophosphate is designed for agricultural use, although some people have used it for home pest control, which is dangerous—and illegal.

Carbamates. This class of compounds includes carbaryl and is similar to organophosphates in that they cause damage to the nervous system. Sevin is one well-known brand that is marketed for use on vegetable gardens.

product is highly toxic, and chronic exposure even at low levels contributes to problems with the nervous system. In fact, chlorpyrifos accounts for most of the pesticide poisonings nationwide. The people most often poisoned are those who work with chlorpyrifos on a regular basis, such as agricultural workers and pesticide applicators, but young children are another very vulnerable group.

You should avoid using any products containing chlorpyrifos or other organophosphates (see "Beware of These Poisons" on page 45 for a list of others). A child's developing nervous system and brain don't need to be exposed to a chemical that can cause this type of damage. Chlorpyrifos and other organophosphate pesticides, even when used according to manufacturer directions indoors, can accumulate on rugs and your child's toys, providing an ongoing exposure to these toxic chemicals.

31 SMART SOLUTION
Get rid of termites safely.

☆☆
Important

△△
Moderately Easy

Organophosphate pesticides are the first choice against termites for most commercial exterminators. (See Smart Solution [30]) Over the past 10 years, chlorpyrifos has been their favorite pick. When the federal ban on most home uses of chlorpyrifos becomes final in 2002, the commercial applicators will probably switch over to diazinon or some other organophosphate—what we like to think of as "playing musical pesticides."

We recommend that instead of resorting to chemical extermination, you consider alternate ways of dealing with termites. According to the National Coalition against the Misuse of Pesticides (NCAMP) in their series of papers, "Least Toxic Control of Pests in the Home and Garden," termites are slow-acting pests—meaning you have a few weeks after you discover them to decide how you want to get rid of them. Here are some nonchemical options.

Extreme heat. A whole house or just a portion of a home can be treated with extreme heat. This method involves exterminators draping the entire roof line of the house or just the area to be treated with a tarp to create a seal; convection heaters with propane burners are set up outside the house and blow hot air through portable ductwork to the infected area inside.

Extreme cold. With this method, exterminators inject liquid nitrogen into the walls of your home where the termites have established their colonies. (A big advantage to this method is that liquid nitrogen can reach termites in otherwise inaccessible areas.)

Electrocution. Termites are electrocuted with a device that releases current through a probe that the exterminator runs over the surface of the wood.

Diatomaceous earth. This mineral kills termites by eroding through their outer shell, causing them to dry up.

Biological controls. Beneficial nematodes (microscopic wormlike creatures) are mixed with water and injected into the soil around your home. Once in the soil, the nematodes seek out and kill the termites.

For more information on nontoxic termite control, see "Resources" on page 145. And remember when considering a professional exterminator to always check the company's references and Better Business Bureau records to make sure the company is reputable.

THE RIGHT QUESTIONS

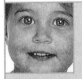

IF YOU do need to call in an exterminator for a pest problem, make sure to ask him the following questions before allowing him to apply any products.

- Are you certified? Most states require pesticide applicators to be certified. Ask to see proof of his certification.

- Do you use Integrated Pest Management (IPM) techniques? If so, what are they? Ask him to be specific.

- What types of chemicals do you use? Request a "material safety data sheet"—which provides chemical names for the pesticides, their toxicity, and potential health effects—for each product used. Be wary if you don't receive any detailed information regarding the types of chemicals used. "Completely safe" pesticides don't exist.

- How often do you think extermination is necessary? The right answer is that regular inspections will be done and pesticides will be applied only when a demonstrated pest problem exists.

- What safer alternatives can you offer?

BEWARE OF CHLORDANE

CHLORDANE, A highly toxic pesticide, was for decades the chemical of choice for termite control. Exterminators drilled holes around the foundation of a house and filled the holes with this chlorinated pesticide. The resulting levels of chlordane in homes were high enough to contaminate the homes and cause long-term health concerns—including cancer.

Chlordane is still measurable at high levels in some homes as long as 35 years after it was applied. If you are buying a home that is more than 10 years old, inquire very carefully as to whether chlordane was ever used in the home. If in doubt, have the house tested for chlordane via a simple air test (contact your state or local health department for recommendations about contractors qualified to perform the test).

Although chlordane was banned in the 1980s, some exterminators still have chlordane in stock. So if you're having your home treated for termites, make sure chlordane won't be used.

32 SMART SOLUTION
Use traps rather than poisons.

Instead of using poison to control ant and roach infestations, try glue traps. Sticky traps contain pheromones that attract these crawling pests. And once the pests step onto the trap, they can't get off.

☆☆
Important

Mechanical traps for getting rid of mice and rodents are also a better choice than using rodent poisons, which are very toxic to children.

△
Easy

33 SMART SOLUTION
Do something about "pesticide drift."

Here's the scenario: Your house windows are open and your children are playing in the backyard with their toys scattered everywhere. A green-and-white truck pulls up in front of your next-door neighbor's house and a lawn maintenance worker in a crisp white uniform unrolls a hose from the truck and starts spraying toxic materials on the lawn next door.

☆☆
Important

△
Easy

A fine chemical mist coats the toys in the yard and your kids. Your kids also inhale the noxious fumes.

The term for what has just happened is called "pesticide drift"—that is, pesticides have wafted from the area where they're being applied. Pesticide drift can expose your family to toxic materials without your knowledge. In fact, studies have shown that some widely used pesticides like chlorpyrifos remain on children's toys for weeks after the initial spraying. Other studies have shown that you can track these chemicals into the house on your shoes—and then small children playing on the floor will inevitably be exposed to them.

You don't have to feel as if your hands are tied, though, when it comes to pesticide drift. Here are a few simple steps to help protect your family from this hazard.

Conduct some neighborly negotiations to remedy the problem. Find out what chemicals are being used on the neighbor's property, then suggest a lawn company that uses nontoxic products, or provide some educational materials on pesticides and safer alternatives.

Contact your local or state health department. Regulations may exist that will help address the problem.

Get your neighbors together to address the problem. (See Smart Solution [81]) Some towns have laws that require that neighbors be notified 48 hours in advance of the application of pesticides on adjoining properties. If you know at least 48 hours in advance, you'll have time to close your windows, bring in the children's toys, and keep the children indoors.

34 SMART SOLUTION
Make peace with your lawn.

A lawn with nary a weed in sight may be a lush, velvety green, but it may also be highly toxic because of all the herbicides that were dumped on it. And the chemicals that you apply to your lawn can end up on your kids when they play in the grass. Those same chemicals also end up in your groundwater as runoff.

☆☆
Important

△
Easy

Instead of competing with the Joneses for the most perfect lawn on the block, learn to tolerate dandelions among your turf. You can also fight lawn weeds the organic, nontoxic way.

Plant the right grass for your region of the country. If you're not sure what type of grass to plant, contact your local cooperative extension office.

Adjust your lawn mower blade to its highest setting. Longer blades of grass will enable the grass to develop stronger root systems and outcompete weeds.

Leave your grass clippings on the lawn. When grass clippings break down, they add valuable nitrogen to the soil, which in turn creates a healthy lawn.

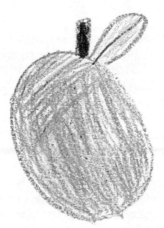

11 Ways to Reduce Exposure to Unsafe Foods

HOW OFTEN do you really pay attention to what goes into your child's mouth? Of course you're on the lookout for that errant penny, paper clip, handful of dirt, or fourth cookie. But we're talking about the meals and snacks you serve him every day. Do you honestly know how healthy all those ingredients are that are listed on a food label? Have you ever thought about the fact that most produce—fruits and vegetables—is sprayed with lots of pesticides?

If you actually take stock of what your child is eating, you might be in for a surprise. That's why we've put together the following 11 points to help you serve your children food that's nutritious *and* safe to eat.

35

SMART SOLUTION
Be fruit and vegetable savvy.

Children need a wholesome diet that includes at least five daily servings of fruits and vegetables. However, the majority of produce available has been sprayed with chemicals, particularly pesticides. In fact, in its landmark report, "Pesticides in the Diets of Infants and Children," the National Academy of Sciences expressed concern that the traces of pesticides found on produce in the diets of infants and children may affect a child's development. And several animal studies have shown that even minuscule amounts

☆☆
Important

△
Easy

of some pesticides—amounts comparable to those found on fruits and vegetables—can interfere with the growth of a child's brain or with the hormones that regulate growth and development. The chemicals that interfere with brain growth are called neurotoxins, and those that interfere with hormones are endocrine disrupters.

Although the jury is still out on the extent to which trace amounts of neurotoxins and endocrine disrupters actually affect a child's growth and development, you should still work to minimize residues of pesticides on the fruits and vegetables you serve your kids. Here are some ways you can do that.

Know which fruits and vegetables have the largest amount of pesticide residues on them. According to a *Consumer Reports* study, apples, grapes, green beans, peaches, pears, spinach, and winter squash had higher toxicity scores than other produce, based on the number of samples with pesticide residues and the toxicity of each pesticide. With this in mind, you might want to limit your child's servings of this produce—and then make sure she eats a variety of the fruits and veggies that have fewer pesticide residues on them.

Clean them up. Scrub and peel fruit and appropriate vegetables (such as carrots) before serving them. Wash greens and oily or waxed soft-skin fruits and vegetables (such as tomatoes) in a mild solution of detergent and water. Rinse well.

Choose certified-organic produce. Organic produce is grown without any synthetic pesticides, herbicides, or fertilizers. Because this food is grown without chemicals, it's free of the toxic residues that are present on traditionally grown (i.e., grown with chemicals) produce.

However, commercial use of the term "organic" has not necessarily followed the intent stated above. Until recently, there was little regulation of the use of the word, and some "organic" produce saw its share of synthetic chemicals. Now, in order for fruits or vegetables to be labeled "organic," they must meet minimum criteria established by the federal government and thus are labeled "certified organic."

Choose locally grown produce, in season. If you can't find organic produce, your next best option is to buy produce that's been grown locally. In general, locally grown fruits and vegetables should not have been treated with as many chemicals as produce grown far away. That's because locally grown produce doesn't need to be picked unripe, ripened with chemicals, and then treated with preservatives for a long cross-country trip.

ACCORDING TO THE ENVIRONMENTAL WORKING GROUP REPORT "OVEREXPOSED: ORGANOPHOSPHATE INSECTICIDES IN CHILDREN'S DIETS," ONE OUT OF FOUR TIMES THAT A CHILD 6 YEARS OLD OR YOUNGER EATS PEACHES, HE IS EXPOSED TO AN UNSAFE DOSE OF **ORGANOPHOSPHATE INSECTICIDES.** (SEE SMART SOLUTION 30)

One tip for making sure you're choosing local produce is to pay attention to what's growing in your area, season by season, and buy it in season. Peas, lettuce, broccoli, asparagus, and spinach are typical springtime vegetables in many parts of the United States. Summer vegetables include tomatoes, peppers, eggplant, squash, cucumbers, and zucchini. Fall vegetables include hard-skinned squashes, such as butternut and winter squash; turnips; potatoes; and onions.

Limit quantities of imported produce. Although most of the produce in this country is grown with the use of chemicals, many dangerous pesticides, such as DDT, have been outlawed because of their long-term toxic effects. Unfortunately, chemical manufacturers have found a marketplace for many now-banned chemicals in countries with less restrictive laws. The pesticides are used in those countries to grow fruits and vegetables that are then imported to the United States. Although our federal government regulates produce imported to this country, there's no doubt that some imported produce with traces of banned pesticides manages to get into our food supply. The best way to tell whether fruits or vegetables are imported is to check the label. If you can't tell from the label, ask your grocer. If he doesn't know where the produce came from, don't buy it.

36
SMART SOLUTION
Stay away from food additives.

Stabilizers, preservatives, emulsifiers, artificial colors and flavorings, food additives to increase shelf life, to make the unripe tomato red, to keep the cracker crisp, to make the cucumber shinier or the broccoli greener, to sweeten without calories or to take the guilt out of potato chips—the myriad food additives in what we eat should give us cause to wonder. Wonder about which are safe; wonder about whether we need them; wonder about whether we should be allowing our children to eat foods containing them.

☆☆
Important

△△
Moderately
Easy

THE SKINNY ON FATS

 WITH OUR society focusing on cholesterol and the dangers of saturated fats, you're wise to consider lowering the level of fats in your family's meals. However, children need some fat, so it's not a good idea to eliminate all fat from their diets. Also be aware that some "fat-free" products substitute excess sugar or dietetic sweeteners for the fat to enhance the product's taste—and those ingredients aren't good choices for your child's diet. A well-balanced diet containing at least five daily servings of fruits and vegetables, some protein, and carbohydrates is ideal.

The short answer is: probably not. The cosmetic enhancements of fresh produce and the hidden ingredients in processed foods may pose a threat to your child's health.

So which food additives should you avoid? Using the theory of prudent avoidance, we suggest that you eliminate as many as possible. This means minimizing exposure to those things that are thought to be linked to health threats, even though the research that can prove or disprove the link may be incomplete or years away. Use your common sense to determine just how much risk you're willing to accept and what level of effort you're willing to commit to avoid items and lifestyles that may prove hazardous to your health or the health of your children.

Although rigorously tested by the federal government, food additives may have long-term health effects that will take years to discover. Sometimes this results in a recall or a ban on a product previously thought to be harmless. For example, cold medications containing phenylpropanolamine hydrochloride were pulled from drugstore shelves across the country because they were found to increase the risk of stroke in young women.

Even if there are no known adverse health effects from a particular food additive, we feel you should limit your child's exposure to it. Fresh food without processing and additives is always preferable to processed food.

Here are some food additives that your child doesn't need.

Saccharin. Studies have shown that saccharin causes cancer in laboratory animals. Although it's approved by the Food and Drug Administration (FDA) for use and is the subject of rigorous quality control, it has no place in the

LIMIT REFINED SUGAR

 ALTHOUGH NOT necessarily thought of as a food additive, re-fined sugar in large quantities has a noticeable effect on the body. After eating a sugar-laden meal, your body's insulin level rises to accommodate the metabolism of the sugar. Parents often describe this as a "sugar high" in their children—when their kids become overactive and irrepressible for a time. Several hours later, the rebound effect occurs and children become sleepy or lethargic. Children whose bodies are growing and developing don't need this cascade of sugar high and rebound lethargy on a daily basis—it increases the risk of obesity and diabetes.

We recommend you limit the use of refined sugars and instead substitute natural fruits and fruit juices for refined sugar. Natural fruits and fruit juices contain sugars that the body metabolizes more slowly than refined sugars, so your children remain on a more even keel during digestion.

diet of a growing child. Few parents would consider using it for their children in the same way they use it for themselves: as a coffee sweetener or a diet dessert ingredient. But are you checking your children's soft drink choices? Encourage your children to avoid diet soda, which may be sweetened with saccharin.

Caffeine. Caffeine is a drug that stimulates the heart, making it beat faster. It also affects the brain by altering the metabolism of brain cells. Caffeine is also mildly addictive, and withdrawal from caffeine can cause irritability and lethargy. All in all, caffeine is no good for a child's developing brain and nervous system. High-caffeine soft drinks such as Jolt and Mountain Dew are the worst caffeine offenders.

Aspartame. This sweetener that comes in the blue packets and in many diet sodas is addictive; it also alters the nervous system by affecting brain receptors and overstimulating the brain. Although the FDA has approved this product for general use, prudent avoidance suggests that you keep it away from your children.

Olestra. Fat-free potato chips? Actually, olestra is an unabsorbable fat that passes through the body without being metabolized. The side effects can include diarrhea, bloating, leakage of stool, and other unpleasantries. Olestra has no place in a child's diet.

37
SMART SOLUTION
Choose organic dairy products.

In 1993, the FDA approved the use of a product called re-combinant bovine somatotrophin (rbST) to increase milk production in dairy cows. This additive increases the level of the hormone IGF-1 in milk. A natural and necessary hor-mone, IGF-1 has also been linked to a number of types of cancer: breast cancer, osteogenic sarcoma (the most common bone cancer in children), colon cancer, and lung cancer. Although research is in its early stages, prudent avoidance indicates that you should avoid serving your chil-dren milk and milk products from cows treated with rbST. Instead, buy milk and milk products that are certified or-ganic because organic dairy farmers can't treat their cows with rbST. If your local grocery store doesn't stock organic milk, ask them to do so. (See Smart Solution 81)

☆☆
Important

△△
Moderately
Easy

38
SMART SOLUTION
Minimize the use of processed foods.

While you don't need to entirely avoid giving your chil-dren processed foods, the "less is more" theory applies here. That's because processed foods may contain ingredients that aren't wholesome—and don't add nutrients to your child's diet. Here are some processed foods to watch out for.

☆☆
Important

△△
Moderately
Easy

Hot dogs, bacon, cold cuts, and other processed meats. These products are all cured with nitrates; during the cooking process, nitrates can be converted into nitrites and nitrosamines, which are carcinogenic. If you barbecue hot dogs until they're black or you burn the bacon, it's more likely that the nitrates will convert into nitrites and ni-trosamines. Since the barbecue process also gives rise to ben-zopyrenes, another cancer-causing substance, a burnt hot dog is high on the list of foods to avoid giving your kids.

Hot dogs and processed meats have also been the sub-jects of multiple major product recalls over the past few years due to a contamination with listeria, a bacterium that can cause pregnant women to miscarry and can cause serious illness in the elderly, infants, and those with im-mune system deficiencies.

Processed cereals. While the addition of nutrients to ce-reals can help assure that your child receives some important vitamins and minerals, most processed cereals contain ex-cess sugar. Also, some processed cereals are made with tropical oils, such as palm or coconut oil. These oils are high in saturated fat, so it's best to avoid them to help prevent cardiovascular disease later in life.

Processed baked goods. Avoid cookies, cakes, and the like made with tropical oils, which are high in saturated fats.

Candy bars. These sweet treats contain caffeine and excess sugar, so minimize the candy habit for your child's sake. Instead, always have plenty of fruit on hand at home, and get your child accustomed to reaching for an apple or a banana (washed or peeled, of course) when he needs a snack.

39 SMART SOLUTION
Cook those burgers well.

Leaving even a bit of pink in your hamburgers when you cook them can spell disaster for your children and for you due to a deadly strain of bacteria—*E. coli* O157:H7— that may be present in hamburger. Case in point: In 1994, hundreds of people in the Seattle area suffered gastrointestinal distress and diarrhea, and several children were afflicted with life-threatening hemolytic uremic syndrome (HUS) after suffering bouts of bloody diarrhea. Health investigators found a common thread relating these tragic events: The children and their families had eaten undercooked hamburgers contaminated with *E. coli* O157:H7 at a fast-food restaurant chain.

☆☆☆
Very Important

△
Easy

Over the next several years, hundreds of other cases of HUS from *E. coli* O157:H7 appeared nationwide—many of which were traced back to undercooked hamburgers.

Why hamburgers? *E. coli* O157:H7 is a bacterium carried naturally in the intestines of cattle. This bacterium may contaminate meat at the slaughterhouse or meat-processing plant when fecal material from the cattle comes in contact with the meat. For those cuts of meat that remain intact during processing, such as steaks, the bacterium tends to remain on the surface of the meat. When you grill or sear the meat, the high temperatures kill the bacterium. So even though you may serve the meat rare—visibly red or pink in the center—*E. coli* O157:H7 may not pose a significant threat because the contamination remained on the outside of the meat and was killed during the frying or grilling.

However, when hamburger is made, the meat is ground. Any contamination present on the outside of the meat is thoroughly mixed into the center of the meat as well. If you cook the meat to only rare, the bacteria in the center aren't killed and can be passed along to the person who eats the rare hamburger.

Because *E. coli* O157:H7 can cause severe illness in kids (they can die from it), it's extremely important that you cook any hamburgers you plan to serve to an internal temperature of 160°F. When burgers are cooked to this temperature, they shouldn't show any pink in the centers. The best way to be sure that the hamburger has reached this temperature is to use an instant-read food thermometer, available at most kitchen-supply stores. You should also teach your children not to eat any hamburgers that are pink in the middle. As an added pre-caution, never place cooked hamburgers back on the same un-washed plate that held the burgers when they were raw.

40 SMART SOLUTION
Buy pasteurized cider.

Cases of *E. coli* O157:H7 (see Smart Solution 39 for the health effects of *E. coli*) have also been linked to unpasteurized apple cider. Small local producers of apple cider often use ap-ples that have fallen to the ground to make their cider. Some-times these apples are contaminated by cow manure that's on the ground. If the contaminated apples aren't thoroughly washed and the apple cider isn't pasteurized, *E. coli* O157:H7 can be passed along in the cider. So, to keep your children safe, make sure the apple cider you're serving them is pasteurized.

☆☆☆
Very
Important

△
Easy

41 SMART SOLUTION
Choose fish wisely.

Our biggest concern about eating fish centers on poly-chlorinated biphenyls, or PCBs, which are now found in some fish. PCBs are manufactured chemicals that were used widely in the production of electrical generators and transformers until their ban in the 1970s. They enter the environment when they are discharged into rivers by industries, as well as from accidental leaks and spills. PCBs were a popular product in industrial settings because they didn't break down easily. That characteristic, though, is why PCBs now appear in places where they were never used or even spilled. Pristine rivers and the far reaches of the Arctic Circle contain traces of PCBs and dioxins (which arise as a result of burning PCBs).

☆☆
Important

△
Easy

PCBs have contaminated a number of waterways in this country, including the Great Lakes and the Hudson River, through industrial runoff and spills. Tiny fish in the waterways consume PCB-contaminated plants and animals. When larger fish, crabs, and lobsters consume the smaller fish that have eaten the contaminated plants, the PCBs become part of the larger fishes' bodies. This process is known as bioaccumulation of PCBs. The larger fish and shellfish in these waters are more contaminated than the smaller fish because they have consumed substantially more PCB-laden fish, whose PCBs become part of the body fat of the larger fish. Eventually, the fisherman catches a fish, and the fish—with its PCBs—becomes part of the person who eats it.

PCB-contaminated fish aren't safe to eat because PCBs can cross the placenta from pregnant mother to baby and are linked to loss of intelligence and problems in behavior. Recent studies of children whose mothers consumed PCB-contaminated fish from the Great Lakes have confirmed these serious problems.

Mercury is another contaminant that moves up the food chain in the same way as PCBs. It, too, is a health problem associated with fish in areas where contamination occurs. In some pristine trout streams and lakes in industrial states, mercury contamination limits the number of fish a person can eat on a weekly or monthly basis. (The FDA sets the limits of contamination allowed in food items, including fish.)

Fish can also become contaminated by chlorinated hydrocarbons, another environmentally persistent chemical. Chlorinated hydrocarbon pesticides such as chlordane and DDT, which were used years ago to treat houses for termites or to kill pests on lawns and gardens, have washed through runoff into some estuaries, streams, and water bodies. Fish become contaminated when they eat the contaminated plants and animals in the water.

While the potential safety issues involved in eating fish are real, we don't want you to keep fish out of your child's diet (or yours). In general, fish are high in essential vitamins and minerals and a wholesome source of protein. You can do a few things, though, to help make sure your kids aren't eating contaminated fish.

- Know where your fish comes from, and don't exceed the recommended frequency for eating fish out of that area.

Contact your state or local health department for a listing of contaminated areas and guidelines for which fish are safe to eat.

- Avoid eating the skin and the fatty layer of fish, which is where PCBs accumulate.

- Choose young, small fish whenever possible because they will contain fewer (if any) toxic contaminants than larger fish.

- Remember that crabs, lobsters, other shellfish, and eels from contaminated waterways can also have high levels of PCBs and other contaminants.

42

SMART SOLUTION
Think twice about peanuts.

☆
Good
Idea

Peanut allergy, a life-threatening allergic reaction, affects between 1 and 1.5 percent of the population. We don't know much about why some children develop this allergy, but some experts think that providing peanut products to children as young as 1 year old may cause them to develop sensitivities that erupt as full-blown peanut allergies later in childhood.

△
Easy

So what, if anything, can you do to help prevent peanut allergy in your children? You may wish to:

Skip the peanut-butter-and-jelly sandwiches for the under-3-year-old crowd. The jury is still out on whether eating peanut butter at an early age triggers later peanut allergies. However, if your child develops a peanut allergy, it has the potential to be deadly.

Avoid peanuts if you're pregnant. Some researchers think peanut allergy may develop later if the fetus is exposed to peanuts via mom while in utero. Again, research on this idea is very preliminary at this time, but you may want to take this prudent avoidance approach.

If your child *is* allergic to peanut products, learn everything you can about how to protect her. You must be extremely cautious that she doesn't eat anything that contains peanuts or peanut oil, as many food products contain one or both of these ingredients. Your pediatrician and local support groups are good places to start for information on protecting your child from exposure.

43 SMART SOLUTION
Choose commercially prepared peanut butter.

Another potential problem with peanuts (and other grains such as corn) is aflatoxin. Aflatoxin is a naturally occurring toxin produced by the mold *Aspergillus flavus*. When this mold contaminates peanuts or corn, it produces a toxin that's passed along to those who eat the peanut or corn products. A child who eats a food product containing high levels of aflatoxin may develop liver failure.

☆
Good
Idea

△
Easy

The good news, though, is that the federal government strictly regulates the amount of aflatoxin that's allowed in food products. Studies by the Consumers Union indicate that the major brands of commercially produced peanut butter (such as Jif, Peter Pan, Skippy, and Smuckers) pass their tests for aflatoxin content with flying colors. (A food scientist at one producer of organic peanut butters, Arrowhead Mills, also assured us that their peanuts are tested regularly for the toxin and they have never found any detectable levels.) However, the studies also show that some fresh-ground peanut butters sold at natural-food stores had levels of aflatoxin that were higher than government standards. Given those findings, we recommend that when buying peanut butter, you choose a well-known brand of commercially prepared peanut butter. If you make your own peanut butter, use roasted top-quality peanuts to make it— roasting may kill the mold that causes aflatoxin.

44 SMART SOLUTION
Grow your own food safely.

Planting and tending a garden is a fun thing for kids to do as well as a great way to provide your family with fresh produce. After all, children need plenty of fruits and vegetables to provide their growing bodies with essential vitamins and minerals.

☆☆
Important

△
Easy

If you're going to plant a garden, though, you need to make sure that you follow some safe practices so that the food you grow isn't contaminated with chemicals. Here are six main points to keep in mind.

Find out the history of the land where you plan to plant. If your neighbors have lived in the area longer than you have, ask them what was there before your house was built. Or check with your local government or health department to be sure the land doesn't have a questionable environmental history. If the land was previously used for an industrial facility, a golf course, or a non-organic orchard, for example, your soil may very well have toxic materials in it.

Don't place your garden too close to the edge of your property. If your house is in an older neighborhood, the outskirts of the property may be teeming with unwanted chemicals that were dumped there (dumping chemicals in the yard was a common practice before the advent of hazardous material drop-off sites). Also, if your garden is next to your neighbor's property, any chemicals he uses on his yard may end up in your garden.

Avoid placing your garden next to a highway or busy street. Runoff from the road can contaminate your garden with chemicals and road salt. Likewise, make sure you plant your garden away from any buildings that have paint chipping off because the paint may contain lead.

Garden organically. When you grow things organically, you don't use any synthetic herbicides, pesticides, or fertilizers. Of course, you might think that not using chemicals would leave your garden open to invasion by weeds and pest insects. But that's not true. Sure, you'll end up with a few weeds and bad bugs here and there, but if you rely on techniques such as amending your soil with compost so it's rich and healthy, your garden will produce a bounty of good things for you and your family to eat. And you'll know that the food you've grown doesn't contain toxins. (For more information on how to garden organically, see "Recommended Reading" on page 144.)

Avoid using pressure-treated lumber. Many gardeners use pressure-treated lumber to define garden beds. The draw of using such lumber is that it stands up to the elements better and lasts longer than lumber that hasn't been treated. However, pressure-treated wood contains arsenic, chromated copper arsenate, and other toxic chemicals. Studies have shown that these chemicals can leach out of the wood and into the soil—meaning those chemicals may, in all likelihood, find their way into your garden produce. If you want to frame your garden beds, use a weather-resistant wood, such as cedar, instead of pressure-treated lumber.

Keep grass clippings that have been treated with pesticides out of your compost pile. And never put dog or cat feces in your compost pile; that waste may contain harmful parasites that could end up in the food you grow.

45 SMART SOLUTION
Make hand washing routine.

We couldn't write this book without stressing the importance of washing hands. And since washing hands and mealtime go together, we thought we'd take the opportunity to mention hand washing here.

If you can get your child to do only one thing to prevent the spread of childhood illnesses and infections, it's washing his hands—washing them before meals, after using the bathroom, after playing with pets, after playing outdoors, after rolling around on the floor, and after blowing his runny nose. Every time.

Hand washing is the single most important public health measure ever devised. It helps prevent diseases that can spread from person to person and from animals to people. It helps tame the spread of the common cold and gastrointestinal upsets.

Proper hand washing, that is. That means two hands lathered with soap and hot water, rubbing vigorously together, as well as scrubbing between the fingers and on the top and back of the hands—all for at least 30 seconds.

☆☆☆
Very
Important

△
Easy

SOAP AND WATER IS BEST

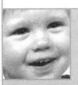

WE DON'T recommend that your children (or you, for that matter) use antibacterial or bacteriostatic hand washes. Good old soap and water is the best choice for routine hand washing.

Germ-killing cleaners are effective in killing most germs, but the germs that they don't kill no longer have to do battle with the more numerous but weaker germs in order to survive. So the stronger germs have an easy playing field on which to grow and multiply. Pretty soon the stronger germs rule the roost. That's how resistant strains of bacteria are encouraged to develop and thrive.

You can help prevent this from happening by not using antibacterial or bacteriostatic cleaners in any form on a routine basis. They're the big guns—save them for real trouble, such as skin infections, or they won't be effective when you need them.

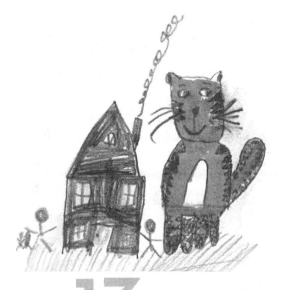

13 Tips for Avoiding Exposure to Household Chemicals

EACH YEAR, poison-control centers across the country receive calls from frantic parents whose children have accidentally ingested toxic chemicals, prescription drugs, and even toxic houseplants. According to the National Safe Kids Campaign (www.safekids.org), in 1997 over 1.1 million accidental poisonings occurred among children under the age of 5 years. The previous year, 109 children younger than 14 were fatally poisoned.

In children 5 years and younger, about 55 percent of poisonings each year are from common household items—cosmetics, cleaning supplies, pesticides, art supplies, and alcohol. Items you probably have in your medicine cabinet—pharmaceuticals and medications—make up 43 percent of poisonings. Given these facts, we can't stress enough how important it is that you take steps to prevent your children from being accidentally poisoned. As you probably know well enough, children are curious—and that curiosity can often lead them down a dangerous path.

Unfortunately, common household items aren't the only things that can poison your children. "Silent" poisons that leach toxic chemicals may exist in your home, too—such as asbestos and radon.

To help protect your child from toxins in the place where he should feel safest—his home—consider the advice on the following pages.

46 SMART SOLUTION
Lock your medicine cabinet.

☆☆☆
Very Important

△
Easy

Locked means locked. Just putting something "up high" isn't good enough—if there's a way for your kids to get to it, they will. Locks also need to be age-appropriate. What keeps a 2-year-old out is not sufficient for a 6-year-old. Of course, although the locks need to be secure enough to thwart your child, they should be easy enough for you to open so that you'll actually use them.

Make sure you lock up both prescription and over-the-counter medications. The contents of both types can spell disaster if your child ingests them.

Here are some of the medications you need to keep secure.

Acetaminophen (Tylenol). Acetaminophen poisoning is extremely serious. Nausea is an early symptom, but after the nausea goes away there's a well-defined lag time of 1 or more days when your child looks fine. Then she can suddenly go into acute liver failure, which can be deadly. A specific antidote for acetaminophen poisoning is available; a child can usually be saved if she is brought to the doctor early and the doctor knows the child has eaten these nonaspirin tablets or liquid. Otherwise, the child can die.

Vitamins with iron. Iron is one of the most toxic substances for children and represents one of the most common types of childhood poisonings. And we're not just talking about adult iron supplements, either. Those yummy-tasting cartoon character or dinosaur-shaped vitamins with fruit candy flavors can just as easily cause iron poisoning. An overdose of iron causes abdominal cramps accompanied by stomach bleeding, followed by a quiet phase when the child seems fine. Then liver toxicity and breakdown of red blood

IF YOU MOVE

MOVING DAY is an especially dangerous time for poisonings. Medications and other poisons that you usually keep securely locked away suddenly are placed in spots where they're accessible to your child. On top of that, your normal household routine is disrupted, making it easy for you to take your eyes off a little one for a few minutes. A good tip for moving day is to always put your medications, cleaners, and other toxic products in a secure place away from your child before the chaos begins.

cells can occur. Like acetaminophen poisoning, iron poisoning can be deadly.

Prescription medicines. If a single dose 1 to 4 times a day is effective in controlling an adult's medical problem, it's likely that a bottle of anything ingested by a child is going to

HIGHLY TOXIC PRODUCTS

THE FOLLOWING table lists common products that you probably have around your house—products that, when ingested in small doses (1 to 2 tablets, capsules, or teaspoonfuls), can be highly toxic to children.

Ingredient	Found In
Acetonitrile	Artificial nail glue
Ammonium fluoride	Rust removers; glass-etching creams; anticavity rinses; wheel cleaners
Benzocaine	Teething gels; vaginal creams, hemorrhoidal creams, first-aid creams
Brodifacoum	Rat poison
Butyrolactone	Super glue solvent
Camphor	Muscle pain creams and ointments
Chloroquine	Antimalarial drugs; arthritis drugs
Chlorpromazine	Thorazine, an antidepressant
Clozapine	Antipsychotic drugs
Desipramine/Tricyclics	Antidepressants; antibedwetting drugs
Diphenoxylate	Antidiarrheal medications
Hydrocarbons	Cleaning fluids; gasoline; kerosene; naphtha
Hyoscyamine	Colic medications
Imidazoline	Eyedrops; nasal decongestants
Lindane	Lice shampoos
Methanol	Glass cleaners; paint strippers; windshield deicers
Methyl salicylate	Over-the-counter liniments, lotions, and food flavorings (oil of wintergreen)
Salt	Seasonings
Selenious acid	Craft compound
Theophylline	Asthma medications

Source: Emery, D., and Singer, J., "Highly Toxic Ingestions for Toddlers: When a Pill Can Kill." Emergency Medicine Reports, 3(12), December 1998.

produce serious to life-threatening results. Treat all prescription medicines as poison and keep them locked up. Never give a child a pill bottle to play with, thinking he can't open it. Also watch what kinds of medicine you keep in your pocket or pocketbook. Those little hands find everything!

Spray antiperspirants. Spray antiperspirants can cause an eye hazard emergency. Sprayed into the child's eye, the antiperspirant irritates the eye and causes pain, redness, and itching. If this happens, flush the eye profusely with water and get to a doctor quickly.

Topical salves. Some of the worst things in the medicine cabinet come in those little tubes that help ease arthritis pain or soothe sunburn. Examples of these products (which are extremely dangerous if your child ingests them) include BenGay and other arthritis medicines; camphor-containing liniments; over-the-counter eyedrops such as Visine, Clear Eyes, and Murine; and anesthetic ointments containing benzocaine, such as Baby Orajel, Anbesol Gel, Lanacane Spray, and Vagisil Creme.

47 SMART SOLUTION
Lock your under-the-sink cabinets.

Of course, the ideal situation is not to keep anything toxic in the cabinets under your kitchen or bathroom sink. If you don't have other options, it's imperative you lock these cabinets. Here are some of the products you use in your home on a regular basis that can contain deadly materials.

Very
Important

Easy

Drain and oven cleaners. These cleaners are extremely toxic materials. It's not worth the risk to have them if you have a child, so get rid of them. (See Smart Solution 17.)

Automatic dishwashing detergent. This product can burn skin and harm eyes; it's toxic if ingested. (Keep in mind that liquid dishwashing detergent poses more of a safety hazard than the powdered kind since a child can drink it.)

Aluminum hubcap cleaners. Hubcap cleaners can contain up to 8 percent hydrofluoric acid, which is highly toxic and can destroy bone.

Furniture oils and waxes. Many of these products are petroleum-based and are toxic.

Kerosene and mineral spirits. These are petroleum-based products and are toxic.

Rug and carpet cleaners. Rug and carpet cleaners usually contain toxic chemicals such as naphthalene.

Industrial-strength cleaners. These cleaners are highly toxic—so don't be tempted to bring a little of the cleaner from work to use in your own home. If you've already brought some home, get rid of it immediately.

Aerosol spray cans. Aerosol cans are linked to a large number of eye injuries, as well as other serious concerns. (See 17)

BE PREPARED

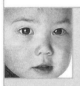

ALTHOUGH WE hope you'll never have to deal with an accidental poisoning in your home, it's always best to be prepared in case of an emergency. This is a good time to remind you to look up the phone numbers of your local poison-control center and fire department or rescue squad—and post them prominently near your phone. Then, check your medicine cabinet and make sure you have syrup of Ipecac on hand. If you don't have any, go out and purchase some (you can get it at any drugstore without a prescription).

Syrup of Ipecac is used to induce vomiting and is often the first line of defense for a child who has been poisoned. But for some poisonings, you *don't* want to induce vomiting. Don't induce vomiting if the substance the child has ingested is caustic (such as a drain cleaner or lye) or has an oily petroleum or hydrocarbon base (such as paint thinners, furniture polish, gasoline, kerosene, or solvents). Always call the poison-control center first because they will tell you what specific steps to take.

When you call poison control, have the product container of the material that caused the poisoning on hand. Be prepared to read the product name and number to the poison control or rescue squad staff. You may be told to give your child syrup of Ipecac. **If you're instructed to go to the nearest hospital, bring the bottle or container that caused the poisoning along with you.** Emergency room physicians tell us that when parents come to the emergency room knowing that their child has eaten something toxic, only 60 percent of the time do they know what the child actually ate. While doctors can run a toxic panel (a blood test to determine what the child has ingested), the toxic panel isn't an instantaneous test, and it picks up only a few substances. By the time the results arrive, valuable time has been lost, during which they could have given the child specific antidotes.

The bottle is also important so the doctors can get the specifics. For example, Tylenol for Cold and Flu is a very different medicine from Tylenol and requires different treatment. Also, the number of pills left in the bottle may help the doctor estimate how much the child ingested. Whether there are one or several types of medicine kept in the same bottle (and you shouldn't keep more than one type of medicine in a bottle) will help the doctor evaluate possible drug interactions.

48

Lock your basement and storage cabinets.

Most basements, garden storage areas, and garages contain a multitude of toxic products that can harm your child. If the products are in a cabinet, you'll certainly want to lock it, but in some instances (such as with a small garden shed) it might be easier if you just lock the front door. Here are some of the items that you'll need to keep out of the hands of your kids.

☆☆☆
Very
Important

△
Easy

Antifreeze. Sweet tasting and toxic, antifreeze is usually made from ethylene glycol and is poisonous if ingested.

Mothballs. Mothballs are made up of a chlorinated, toxic compound and are a suspected carcinogen. Mothballs are particularly appealing to children because they look like candy. We recommend that you avoid using mothballs and try a nontoxic alternative instead. An old-time approach that works quite well is to store your clothes in an airtight container along with cedar blocks.

Paints, lacquers, thinners, and automotive chemicals. All of these solvents can be toxic if inhaled or ingested. And some latex paints contain mercury compounds that can release toxic mercury vapor into room air as the paint dries. So avoid paints with mercury or other toxic chemicals added to the paint to kill mildew. (See Smart Solution 53)

Pesticides. These products are toxic and potentially deadly. (See 29–34)

Photographic and hobby chemicals. Chemicals used for developing photos and other hobbies often contain volatile solvents or heavy-metal pigments. For example, oil paint contains cadmium, lead, chromium, and other heavy metals. Cadmium causes lung and kidney damage. At low levels, lead can damage a child's learning potential; at higher levels, it can cause seizures and neurological system damage.

LOCK UP THAT LIQUOR

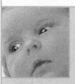
EVEN THOUGH having liquor in your home isn't as dangerous as having a gun, the lure of the forbidden makes alcohol a double threat. Lock liquor cabinets securely to prevent toddlers from ingesting toxic quantities of alcohol—and lock them even more securely to prevent adolescent children and teens from experimenting with alcohol and possibly causing toxic overdoses or alcohol-related injuries. A better preventative would be to not keep alcohol in your home.

GUNS AND KIDS DON'T MIX

ALTHOUGH GUNS are more of a "safety" issue than a "toxic" one, we feel so strongly about them that we wanted to give them some attention in this book. In 1997, firearms caused 32,426 deaths in the United States. According to the Centers for Disease Control and Prevention, injuries from firearms were the second leading cause of death in 1994 for young people between 10 and 24 years of age. And between 1985 and 1994, the risk of dying from a firearm injury more than doubled for teenagers 15 to 19 years of age.

Statistics also tell us that if you keep a gun in your house to protect your family, a bullet from that that gun is more likely to end up killing your child or a neighbor's child than an intruder. A gun in the house is a major child health hazard. As public health professionals, we strongly recommend that you *don't* keep guns in your house if you have children.

However, we do realize that in some special instances, such as in the case of police officers, a gun may be kept at home. In these situations, the gun owner must accept the enormous 24-hour-a-day burden and responsibility to ensure that the gun does not injure or kill a child.

If you must keep a gun, take every precaution you can to keep your gun secure. You must never let down your guard. Never store a loaded gun, and don't store the gun with the bullets. Use a tamperproof lock and keep control of the key. But most importantly, know that children are more skilled at outwitting you than any perpetrator of crime—and they're also curious.

Teaching your children about gun safety is admirable, but it's not a solution to the problem of unintentional gun injuries. Your child is just a child; his friends are just children. You are the one who is ultimately responsible for protecting your child from injury.

SMART SOLUTION

49 Use alternatives to toxic cleaners.

☆☆
Important

Easy

Those antibacterial, germ-killing, sterilizing sprays and wipes that are so popular these days simply aren't worth it. No matter how much of that stuff you use, you'll rarely achieve a "germ-free" kitchen or bathroom. In fact, it's both impractical and unnecessary to try to sterilize your kitchen, your bathroom, or the air you breathe. When you use toxic cleaners you're just substituting a chemical hazard (the cleaners) for a biological hazard (the germs). Plus, overusing germ killers can actually help encourage the growth and development of "superbugs" that resist the germ killer. (See Smart Solution 45)

FOR A **NONTOXIC OVEN CLEANER,** WARM THE OVEN, MOISTEN THE DIRTY PARTS WITH WATER, THEN SPRINKLE THEM WITH BAKING SODA AND SCRUB WITH STEEL WOOL UNTIL THEY'RE CLEAN.

Instead of trying to achieve a *sterile* environment for your kitchen or bathroom, work toward achieving a *clean* environment by using fewer toxic products. Concentrated multipurpose green (environmentally friendly) soaps such as Simple Green, diluted as directed on the package, work well for most purposes. (See "Resources" on page 145 for companies that sell environmentally friendly cleaning products.) If you need to disinfect a countertop, dilute ¼ cup of household bleach in 1 gallon of water and use that mixture. (Before using, test the solution on a small area to make sure it doesn't damage the surface or affect the color.)

50 SMART SOLUTION
Buy in small quantities.

From time to time, you may find it necessary to buy a product that contains a toxic ingredient—such as a caustic drain cleaner if your sink becomes badly clogged or some oily furniture polish to spiff up the dining room table the day before an important party. When that's the case, buy the smallest amount you need to do the job, and then safely dispose of any leftovers immediately after you've finished. That way, you won't have any half-full containers for your child to get into.

☆ Good Idea

△ Easy

51 SMART SOLUTION
Do an annual household chemical inventory.

Spring and fall cleaning are time-honored rituals. Time to take down the curtains and wash the windows, dust behind the hard-to-move furniture, and move the refrigerator to wipe up all those crumbs that have accumulated underneath. Clean up, paint up, fix up. Another important item to add to your to-do list, though, is to take stock of all the chemicals you have in your house and then throw away what you can do without.

☆ Good Idea

△ Easy

The first thing you need to do is to find out how to get rid of unwanted household chemicals in your neighborhood. Many communities have annual "Household Chemical Cleanup" days when you can bring household

HIDDEN DANGERS

OLDER HOUSES may have some very dangerous chemicals stored in those dark, dank cubbyholes in the basement, attic, or garage. If you're a new homeowner and come across an area that has unlabeled containers of chemicals—or containers that seem to be in poor condition and have drips or emit fumes—leave the containers alone and contact your local fire department immediately. Some chemicals, such as ethers and picric acid, are highly explosive if they've aged and become crystalline. Others, such as mercury, are toxic and need professional cleanup. *Never* attempt to clean up a toxic chemical yourself.

chemicals to a central location where they'll be removed and disposed of properly. Check with your local government or trash disposal service for scheduled clean-up days in your area. Most often, these events are held in spring or fall. Time your inventory and collection of unwanted chemicals to take advantage of this activity. If your town doesn't have such days, include this as a useful activity for Smart Solution 81.

When looking through your home for old chemicals, make sure to thoroughly check out these areas.

Basement. Look for old paints, varnishes, oils, cleaners, spot removers, photographic chemicals, automotive chemicals, strippers, and solvents. Get rid of all the ones you absolutely don't need—and then make sure to lock up the ones you feel you need to keep.

Garage and garden storage. Look for containers of pesticides, fertilizers, antifreeze, lawn-mower oil or fuel, and charcoal lighter fluid. If you need to keep any of them, you need to lock them up.

Under the kitchen sink. Look for glass cleaners, floor polishes, drain cleaners, waxes, floor cleaners, jewelry cleaners, furniture polishes, bleaches, dishwashing detergent, and counter cleaning preparations. Again, properly dispose of anything you don't need, and keep what you do need in a safe (locked) place.

Bathroom medicine chest. Look for bottles of rubbing alcohol, hydrogen peroxide, beauty products, and expired medications (both prescription and over-the-counter). Keep only what's necessary in a safe place.

52 SMART SOLUTION
Get rid of unwanted chemicals safely.

Important

Moderately
Easy

For too many years, a corner of the backyard has been a convenient disposal site for used automobile oil, leftover antifreeze, and the last few ounces of turpentine, gasoline, or herbicide. The storm drain in the street has served as a place to pour detergent solution used to wash the car.

At first glance, these seem like small things. But the amount of materials disposed of in our backyards and our storm drains adds up. Products such as oil, gasoline, and antifreeze contain toxic materials that, disposed of carelessly in the backyard or down storm drains, can get into wells, streams, lakes, and groundwater—and then end up in our drinking water. They can also end up on our children when they play outside on contaminated dirt.

Your backyard, garage, attic, and basement are no place to discard unwanted chemicals. You shouldn't put them out with your regular trash for pickup or throw them in trash dumpsters, either.

Instead, contact your local government or trash collection service to find out what you should do with such materials. Some communities have established household chemical cleanup days. If your town has one, take advantage of it. If not, why not consider getting one set up?

53 SMART SOLUTION
Choose paint wisely.

Important

△
Easy

Although the interior water-based paints on the market today are less toxic than latex paint produced years ago, they still contain ingredients that can pose health problems. For example, some kitchen and bathroom paints are advertised as "mildew resistant." These often contain mercury, a toxic metal, which acts as a fungicide. Avoid these paints, as well as any others that claim to contain fungicides. Instead, kill mildew on the surface to be painted by using a dilute solution of chlorine bleach in water (¼ cup bleach to 1 gallon of water). After painting, keep the room well ventilated to prevent the growth of mildew.

All paints contain solvents that evaporate over a period of days as the paint "cures." (See Smart Solution [17]) So make sure to air your house out frequently during the first few days and weeks after painting to minimize the exposure to solvents.

54

SMART SOLUTION
Do your refinishing projects outside.

☆☆
Important

△
Easy

Have you found yourself the heir to old family furniture? You know—those chairs that were once lovely and now are covered with layers of paint, or chests of drawers that have old and crumbling varnish. Of course you'll want to keep these treasures—you just need to refinish them and give them a brand-new look.

Keep in mind, though, that nearly all of the products used to refinish furniture contain toxic materials. The most dangerous of these is methylene chloride. It vaporizes readily and can cause severe damage to the liver and blood-producing systems of the body, which is why we stress that you avoid using any products that contain it. (See Smart Solution 17)

And when you strip furniture, do so outdoors. With adequate ventilation, you can minimize not only your exposure to the toxic ingredients in paint strippers but your child's exposure, as well.

It is extremely important that you never remove paint with a heat gun or blowtorch. Assume that any old paint on furniture or household woodwork contains lead, unless proven otherwise. Lead paint was used extensively on furniture and on both interior and exterior woodwork prior to 1970. Lead has a low melting point and vaporizes readily when heated, and the surest way to get lead poisoning is to inhale vaporized lead paint. Some of the highest blood lead levels in adults and children are seen in families that have used heat guns, hair dryers, or blowtorches to remove lead paint. (See 21)

55

SMART SOLUTION
Have your house tested for radon.

☆☆☆
Very
Important

△△
Moderately
Easy

Radon is an invisible gas produced by the natural radioactive decay of uranium in the earth. In many parts of the country, rocks containing uranium produce radon gas that percolates up through the soil and into the basements of homes, schools, and businesses.

In some areas, levels of radon gas found in homes are high enough to cause health problems. It's estimated that radon gas causes over 10,000 lung cancer deaths annually in the United States.

Because radon is a gas, it migrates readily from the ground into the basements of buildings through cracks in the foundation, in gaps around household piping, and in well water. The amount of radon that enters a building depends upon the underlying rock foundations in the area and the specific configuration of foundation cracks and air pressure within the house. When radon exists deep in the ground in your area, the intake vents for the hot-air heating system or whole-house roof exhaust fans can draw it into the house. Any situation that causes lower air pressure in the basement than in the outside air can bring radon into the house.

To find out if your house has radon, you'll need to have a radon test done. You can have your house tested for radon by a professional, or you can purchase a radon kit at your local hardware store or through your local or state health department and test for radon yourself.

If you decide to do it yourself, you'll have two options when it comes to kits: a charcoal-based kit or an alpha-tracker. A charcoal-based kit is designed for short-term use. It gives a quick indication of how much radon is accumulating over a few days or a week. An alpha-track detector is designed to measure radon over longer periods of time—up to 12 months. Since radon levels in a house can vary over time, this detector generally gives more accurate results than the charcoal-based one, but you have to wait longer for an answer.

RADON REVELATION

RADON WAS only recently identified as a hazard. In 1984, a construction engineer who lived in a small town in Pennsylvania entered the nuclear power plant in Limerick, Pennsylvania, where he was working, and he set off all of the radiation detectors. His home in Berks County was tested for radiation, where it was found to have a radiation level of 2,700 pCi/l, due to radon. This level was higher than any previously measured home in the United States. The engineer and his family were advised to leave their home immediately until radon levels could be brought back to normal.

The high levels of radiation were caused by radon seeping into his home from the rock formations in the area. The region of the country known as the Reading Prong, an area of the Appalachian Mountains that spans from Pennsylvania to New Jersey to New York, is one of the hot spots for radon in this country. Other hot spots are found in some areas of New England and in the intermountain West where uranium is mined. However, radon can be found to some degree in rock formations throughout North America.

Both kits will give you a reading of the quantity of radon in your house in units of picocuries per liter of air (pCi/l). To figure out how concerned you should be about the levels of radon in your house, refer to the following EPA guidelines.

Level of Radon	What You Should Do
More than 200 pCi/l **Extremely high/ Immediate danger**	Follow up immediately, using an alpha-track detector, for no longer than 1 week. If you get the same results, call a qualified radon abatement contractor as soon as possible. You may need to leave your house until the problem is solved.
20–200 pCi/l **Very high**	Rapid follow-up needed. Use an alpha-track detector, exposing it for no longer than 3 months. If the test results are still 20–200 pCi/l, call in a qualified radon abatement contractor and have the problem taken care of as soon as possible.
4–20 pCi/l **High**	Use an alpha-track detector, exposing it for 1 year. If the results are still 4–20 pCi/l, call in a qualified radon abatement contractor.
Less than 4 pCi/l **Acceptable**	Your home has very little or no radon in it. Stay up-to-date about radon recommendations, though, in case they change in the future.

If you have unsafe levels of radon in your home, your best course of action is to hire a trained radon abatement contractor. You can get lists of certified radon inspectors from your state or local health department or from the EPA's 10 regional offices. Before you sign a contract, however, make sure you have answers to these questions, and make sure you check his references.

- Does the contractor have a certificate of his qualifications? Ask to see it.

- Has the contractor surveyed the property and submitted a detailed plan of action, with an estimate?

- How many homes has he remediated? What methods has he used? Is his work guaranteed?

A radon abatement contractor may take a variety of measures to correct the radon problem in your home. His first priority will be finding out how the radon is getting in, so he'll check your drains, cracks in basement walls, and your water supply. Some of the short-term control measures he may take include opening windows, blowing outdoor air into the house with a window fan, and venting crawl spaces. Long-term measures include pumping air into the basement and sealing radon entry routes.

If you're thinking about turning a basement room into living quarters, a den, or a playroom, make sure you have it tested for radon first. And if you need to do major renovations, ask your contractor about using techniques to minimize radon levels in the room over the long term. Keep in mind that construction can change radon levels, so retest your house for radon after the construction is completed.

56 SMART SOLUTION
Have your home checked for asbestos.

We discuss asbestos in more detail in Smart Solution 74, but we want to touch on some of the important points here. Asbestos is a white mineral that was used extensively (until the early 1970s) in households for its fire-retardant properties. Very old furnaces and pipes were covered with thick, white, bandage-like asbestos to prevent furnace fires and heat loss. Researchers think that the reason asbestos causes cancer is that it sheds particles so tiny that you can inhale them deep into your lungs. Because your lungs can't clear the particles, they act as focal spots for cancers to develop. Both lung cancer and mesothelioma, a type of cancer associated almost exclusively with asbestos exposure, can result.

☆☆
Important

△△
Moderately Easy

Asbestos has also been extensively used in roofing shingles, floor tiles, and auto brake linings. It's found in some brands of play sand, as well. (Check the label to make sure it doesn't contain tremolite, a form of asbestos. If it's not labeled tremolite-free, don't buy it.)

If you're not sure whether you have asbestos in your home, contact a certified contractor for an evaluation. Ask the contractor to show you proof of his certification.

The contractor should be able to:

- Show you his asbestos license or training certificate

- Point out areas in your home where he'll need to remove or encapsulate asbestos

- Test questionable material

- Provide documentation showing that the asbestos will be taken to an approved landfill or disposal area

- Avoid dispersing asbestos fibers outside the work area through encapsulation of the area

- Prevent asbestos from getting into the air circulation system of your house

57 SMART SOLUTION
Keep insulation off limits.

Fiberglass insulation is widely used in homes these days. In fact, you may have some extra rolls stored in your attic or basement. While fiberglass looks soft and fluffy, you definitely don't want your children playing with it for two main reasons.

First, fiberglass is glass. The fibers cut, scratch, and can irritate skin. Second, the tiny particles that break off fiberglass are suspected of causing health problems in a fashion similar to asbestos, although not as severe. Because we're still not sure whether fiberglass causes long-term respiratory problems, we advise you to not let your kids play in it and to keep any insulation that you haven't yet installed in a plastic bag or other wrapper so that it doesn't shed particles into your basement or attic.

☆☆
Important

△
Easy

58 SMART SOLUTION
Give away your toxic houseplants.

Some of the most beautiful houseplants are actually quite toxic. Since houseplants aren't usually amenable to being kept in locked cabinets, how about finding new homes for the following in households without children?

☆☆
Important

△
Easy

BOTANICAL NAME	COMMON NAME
Alocasia spp.	Elephant's ears
Aloe vera	Aloe
Amaryllis spp.	Amaryllis
Caladium spp.	Angel wings
Chrysanthemum spp.	Chrysanthemums
Cyclamen spp.	Cyclamens
Dieffenbachia spp.	Dumb cane
Epipremnum aureum	Golden pothos
Euphorbia pulcherrima	Poinsettias
Philodendron spp.	Philodendrons

PART TWO

PROTECTING YOUR CHILD IN YOUR NEIGHBORH

AN ENVIRONMENTAL CHECKLIST FOR YOUR NEIGHBORHOOD

Because your child spends so much time at home, you've probably done as much as you can to make your house a safe haven for him. But what happens when he goes to day care or school—or is just playing a block away at the park? How safe is he from environmental toxins when he's not under your roof?

To find out what areas of your neighborhood might harbor potential environmental hazards, read through this checklist, answering the questions as you go. As you answer, check the numbers (if any) that follow your responses. Those numbers correspond to the numbered "Smart Solutions" throughout this book that can help you prevent or eliminate the unsafe situation.

AT DAY CARE

The boxed numbers indicate which SMART SOLUTION(s) you should review.

Do you have an infant or preschool child who is or will be cared for OUTSIDE YOUR HOME?
○ Yes 59 60 61 62 63 68   ○ No

Does your day care use PESTICIDES?
○ Yes 67   ○ No   ○ Don't know 67

Has there been a problem with HEAD LICE in your day care?
○ Yes 65   ○ No

Does your day care apply INSECT REPELLENT to children when outdoors?
○ Yes 70   ○ No

Have you checked on the FIRE SAFETY of your day care?
○ Yes   ○ No 59

Does your day care use toxic CHEMICALS or CLEANERS?
○ Yes 63 68   ○ No

(continued)

The boxed numbers indicate which SMART SOLUTION(s) you should review.

Is there an OUTDOOR play area at your child's school or day care?
○ Yes 68   ○ No

Have you checked on whether your day care meets HEALTH STANDARDS?
○ Yes   ○ No 60 64

AT SCHOOL

Do you have a SCHOOL-AGE child?
○ Yes 71 72 73 74 75 77
○ No

Is there a PTO (Parent Teacher Organization) or PTA (Parent Teacher Association) at your child's school?
○ Yes   ○ No 71

Does the PTO or PTA have a group that reviews ENVIRONMENTAL issues?
○ Yes 71   ○ No 71

Has the environmental issues group reviewed the potential environmental HAZARDS around the school?
○ Yes   ○ No 76

Has your school been INSPECTED for asbestos, lead paint, and lead in drinking water?
○ Yes   ○ No 74 75
○ Don't know 74 75

Does your school have SCIENCE LABS?
○ Yes 77   ○ No

Does the school have written procedures about how to handle hazardous SPILLS?
○ Yes   ○ No 71 79

IN YOUR NEIGHBORHOOD

Have you lived in the same NEIGHBORHOOD all your life?
○ Yes   ○ No 82

Have you surveyed your neighborhood recently for environmental HAZARDS?
○ Yes   ○ No 82

Do you know what industrial CHEMICALS are released into your community?
○ Yes 90   ○ No 84 90

Do you know the SOURCE of your drinking water?
○ Yes   ○ No 83

Does your community use ROAD SALT for deicing in the winter months?
○ Yes 86   ○ No

Do you belong to a community group that works on ENVIRONMENTAL issues?
○ Yes   ○ No 81 84

Has your community taken a stand against EXCESSIVE fertilizer and pesticide usage?
○ Yes   ○ No 84 85

12 Hints for Averting Day Care Hazards

FINDING THE right caregiver for your child outside your home can be a challenge. After all, your child is your most precious gift—you can't leave her with just anyone. So no matter what sort of care you choose—whether it's leaving your child at Grandma's house or at a licensed day care— you'll want to make sure the building where she'll be staying is safe from environmental hazards. Here are some of the most important things to keep in mind.

59 SMART SOLUTION
Make sure your day care meets fire safety codes.

Fire safety codes for licensed day cares are regulated by law. The law requires that nonflammable construction materials are used, emergency exits are available, smoke alarms are installed, and each staff member is properly trained for a fire emergency. Having your child stay in a building with fire regulations is a benefit because the regulations add a measure of protection your child may not get in an unlicensed facility. People who die in fires usually don't die from the fire itself but from inhaling fumes produced by burning toxic materials. So if your day care facility meets fire codes, your child is less likely to be exposed to the life-threatening toxic products that result from a fire.

Depending on where you live, many agencies may be involved in regulating licensed day care, such as the state department of social services or the education department.

☆☆
Important

△
Easy

Whenever multiple agencies are responsible for the regulation of a facility, you'll have definite benefits. Many sets of eyes make it less likely that a serious problem will go unaddressed. But the risk that something will slip through the cracks still exists. That's why it's always a good idea to make your own assessment of how well the licensed day care facility is doing. You should ask the provider:

- When the facility was last inspected by the fire department

- If you can see the results of each inspection

- If the renewal of the permit requires a visit by the fire inspector or just a paper submission

Double-check the answers with the regulating agency for details on what is covered under the fire department regulations and under the other applicable code regulations.

Of course, your child might receive care outside your home in a place like Grandma's house, which doesn't have a formal licensing requirement. In that case, you have more of a burden to make sure your child is safe from toxic materials, as well as from the risks of fire.

Be objective when you review the place where you leave your child. Just because someone is a family member or a close friend doesn't mean that there aren't any toxins or other environmental hazards around. So get a checklist from your local fire department and perform a fire safety check of the house yourself. (If you don't feel comfortable doing that, suggest to the homeowner that a review of his home by the local fire department would be worthwhile.) Here are some fire hazards to look for.

Extension cords. Look for fraying, many things plugged into the same outlet, or cords strung out around the room. Too many cords may indicate an outdated electrical system that can become overloaded and cause a fire.

Gasoline or kerosene room heaters. These heaters are highly flammable. In addition, their vapors can accumulate in confined areas and ignite with explosive results. If the heaters tip over and spill fuel, you could end up with a fire or explosion on your hands. Because gasoline and kerosene room heaters are so dangerous, they shouldn't be used.

Improper indoor storage. Be on the alert for piles of newspapers in the cellar or attic, flammable materials stored indoors, and propane tanks or gasoline kept inside the house (which is *extremely* dangerous).

Smoke hazards. Ask if the chimney, furnace, and hot-water heater are cleaned on a regular basis. Find out about cigarette smoking, as well. Do caregivers smoke indoors? Are burning cigarettes ever left unattended? (Remember, no child should be exposed to tobacco smoke.)

When reviewing the home for fire safety, don't forget to check the exit routes from the house. Ask yourself the following questions.

- Are the doors accessible and easily opened, or are they blocked by furniture?

- Does each floor of the house have several escape routes?

- Do the windows open easily?

- Does everyone in the house know how to escape from any room in the house in case of fire?

- Are there fire escape ladders available in the upper floors of the house? Are they long enough to reach the ground?

- Do household residents know where to meet outside the house in case of fire so the firefighters will know if someone is trapped inside?

Finally, check to make sure the home contains fire extinguishers and smoke detectors and that they're up-to-date and in working order. Make sure the members of the home know how to use them properly.

60 SMART SOLUTION
Make sure your day care meets health codes.

Ask your local health department for guidance on how to be sure that a day care facility is protected against health risks. Some possible environmental hazards you'll want to check for include lead paint (indoors and out) and pesticide use. (See Smart Solutions 61 67)

☆☆
Important

△
Easy

Sanitation is another area you'll want to investigate, as children can spread not only germs but also toxic materials through poor sanitation. Make sure all the toilets work and that there aren't any problems with the septic system. Look in each bathroom to see that it's clean and that there is soap available for hand washing. And, of course, make sure every person is washing his hands after using the bathroom. (See 45)

61 SMART SOLUTION
Be sure your day care is "lead safe."

Lead poisoning is a danger to children, especially to children under the age of 6 years, whose brains and nervous systems are developing. (See Smart Solutions ⓳–㉘ for more information on lead paint and its relationship to childhood lead poisoning.) That's why it's really important that your day care doesn't have lead paint problems.

☆☆☆
Very
Important

△△
Moderately
Easy

Lead paint was widely used in buildings built before 1970. Use the same guidelines recommended for your home (See ⓳) to be sure that your day care is not a source of lead poisoning for your child. Remember that Grandma's house is as likely to have lead paint as any other type of day care facility built before 1970. You may have lived in the house as a child and had no problems but like you, the lead paint in your childhood home is much older now and may be chipping in places that only a child can find.

62 SMART SOLUTION
Make sure medications are locked up.

You, like most parents out there, have probably sent your child to day care along with a bottle of cough suppressant or the prescription antibiotics that she needs to finish. And while medications can certainly help make an ill child better, an overdose of medication can make a healthy child very sick. (See Smart Solution ㊻)

☆☆☆
Very
Important

△
Easy

So check the day care to make sure that all medications are locked away and stored out of reach of children.

63 SMART SOLUTION
Insist on nontoxic cleaners.

Many common household cleaners contain toxic ingredients that you don't want your child exposed to. (See Smart Solution ㊾) After these cleaners are used, traces of them can remain on tabletops, carpets, floors, and toys in your day care center. When your child crawls on the floor or puts toys in his mouth, he may ingest traces of the cleaner. When these cleaners are used properly, exposure to their residues is a minimal risk. Still, accidental ingestion of some of these products can be life threatening.

☆☆
Important

△
Easy

In her book *Clean and Green*, Anne Berthold-Bond outlines hundreds of alternatives to toxic commercial cleaners. She also reports the results of her survey of the chemicals found in commercial products—and their health impacts. Here is a sampling of the products and health effects she cites, as well as some recommendations for using the cleaners.

Commercial All-Purpose Cleaners

- These may contain phosphates, which cause algae blooms that deplete water of oxygen. Phosphates also cause water pollution when they get into lakes, bays, and rivers.

- Chlorinated compounds in cleaners don't break down easily and become persistent in the environment. They are also stored in fat cells and can be passed to children via a nursing mom's breast milk.

- Petroleum-based products in cleaners also do not break down and are persistent in the environment, contaminating our water and air.

- Other dangerous substances found in cleaners can include glycol ether, Stoddard solvent, naphtha, and kerosene. These are all neurotoxins that can cause headaches and confusion with overexposure.

- Oven and drain cleaners are especially dangerous. They contain corrosive lye and cause severe burns of the throat if swallowed by a child.

Recommendations

- Avoid commercial cleaners described with these warning words: caution, danger, corrosive, or caustic.

- Try a sampling of products from some of the companies that produce least-toxic products (such as Seventh Generation, Ecover, and Lifetree).

- Use plain soap and water for most cleaning projects.

- If you need to disinfect an area after a spill of infectious material, do so using a dilute solution of chlorine bleach in water (¼ cup household bleach to 1 gallon of water).

Commercial Deodorizers

Commercial deodorizers can contain some dangerous chemicals, including methoxychlor, petroleum distillates, formaldehyde, p-dichlorobenzene, and naphthalene. All of these chemicals are toxic, so avoid unnecessary exposure.

Recommendations

• Avoid using commercial deodorizers, including the plug-in type.

• Keep the air fresh by cleaning up spills promptly and airing out the room.

Commercial Disinfectants

• Naphtha is a petroleum mixture. Exposure in large quantities can cause dizziness or other central nervous system symptoms when inhaled.

• Some components of petroleum mixtures, such as benzene, have been shown to cause cancer. Ingestion of petroleum mixtures are also toxic.

• Chlorinated germicides contain chlorinated compounds, many of which are persistent in the environment and can accumulate in the body, with the potential to cause adverse health effects.

• Sodium sulfite can cause severe respiratory distress, especially in people with asthma.

Recommendation

• When you need to disinfect something occasionally (such as when a child is sick with an infectious disease), use a dilute solution of chlorine bleach in water (¼ cup household bleach in 1 gallon of water).

Dishwasher Detergents

Automatic dishwasher detergents can contain petroleum-based surfactants, naphtha, germicides, chloro-o-phenylphenol, and sodium nitrites (which cause ingestion problems).

Recommendations

• Choose a dishwashing detergent that is phosphate free. Also note that dishwashing detergents contain the word "caution" on their label and should always be kept out of reach of children.

• Consider using products developed by manufacturers that specialize in least-toxic products.

• Make sure the dishes are well rinsed before they're used.

Toilet Cleaners

These are among the most toxic materials used for routine cleaning. They may contain sodium acid oxalate, o-dichlorobenzene, fungicides, and chlorinated phenols—all of which are highly toxic.

Recommendations

- Use a borax solution to clean the inside of the toilet bowl.

- Mix a solution of equal parts white vinegar and water to clean the toilet rim (the part where children come into contact with the toilet).

Carpet Cleaners

Most carpet cleaners contain powerful allergens. (See [13])

Recommendations

- Use washable rugs instead of installed wall-to-wall carpeting when feasible. (See [13])

- Choose least-toxic carpet cleaners from a manufacturer that makes least-toxic cleaner alternatives.

64 SMART SOLUTION
Be a hand-washing monitor.

Hand washing by both children and caregivers is vital in preventing kids from ingesting toxic materials (such as lead dust or contaminated soil) and in decreasing the spread of communicable diseases. Of course, the chances of ingesting toxic materials or spreading diseases are reduced when kids and caregivers practice not just good, but *great* hand-washing techniques. (See Smart Solution [45])

☆☆ Important

△ Easy

Check to make sure that day care workers wash their hands:

- After using cleaners or products containing chemicals

- Before preparing food

- After changing an infant's diaper

- After wiping a runny nose or cleaning up other infectious materials

- After using the toilet

Also encourage day care workers to wash tabletops, toys, changing tables, and common areas frequently. Soap and water works well. A mild bleach solution—¼ cup household bleach to 1 gallon of water—is even better for sanitizing most heavily used surfaces.

Children need to wash their hands, too (we recommend supervised hand washing up to the age of 4 to 6 years old, depending on how well the child can wash her hands by herself). They should always wash their hands:

- After playing outside
- Before eating
- After using the toilet
- After playing with pets

ANIMALS AND DISEASE

 THE ISSUE of animals and disease doesn't really fall into the category of chemical toxins, but it is an environmental hazard, so to speak. You should be aware of three serious diseases that can be spread through contact with animals: salmonella, rabies, and *E. coli* O157:H7.

Salmonella is an intestinal disease carried by reptiles and amphibians, and it can be transmitted to people. Because reptiles slither around in their droppings, salmonella may end up on their skin. If your child touches a reptile that has salmonella on its skin and then puts his unwashed hand in his mouth, he may end up with salmonella (which can cause serious illness in children). So encourage staff members at day care to find new homes for any snakes, lizards, or turtles that are current residents.

Rabies is another serious disease found in some animals—including bats, skunks, raccoons, foxes, and other wildlife. It's spread through the saliva of the infected animal. If a person is bitten or scratched by a rabid animal, she will need rabies shots to prevent contracting this disease, which is fatal.

Most people in the United States who die from rabies contracted it from a bat. If a bat is found at day care, neither the children nor the staff members should handle it and it must be presumed to be rabid.

E. coli O157:H7 is a bacterium that can cause potentially life-threatening illness, particularly in children. This bacterium is present in the intestines of cattle; most people who contract *E. coli* O157:H7 do so by eating undercooked hamburger made from contaminated meat. (See 39) However, there have been documented cases of *E. coli* O157:H7 infection from other sources, such as in children who have touched infected animals at petting zoos, and from unpasteurized apple cider.

To help prevent an *E. coli* O157:H7 infection in your child, make sure he washes his hands thoroughly after contact with animals. Also, always serve hamburger that has been cooked to an internal temperature of 160°F, and serve only pasteurized fruit juices.

65 SMART SOLUTION
Treat head lice nontoxically.

Hearing for the first time that your child has head lice invokes everything from dread and revulsion to embarrassment and panic in many parents. Until it happens to your family, you can't fully appreciate the misery of a child with head lice.

☆☆
Important

△△△
Difficult

One fateful day, the letter comes home from day care:

> Dear Parent:
> I regret to inform you that the school nurse has identified your child as having head lice. It is necessary that you do the following things before your child will be readmitted to the class:
> 1. Purchase a special shampoo for head lice from your local pharmacy; make sure your shampoo comes with a special "nit comb" to remove "nits"—the tiny, waxy egg sacs that attach to the hair shafts. Purchase enough for every family member.
> 2. Inspect every family member's hair for head lice and have everyone in the household wash his hair with the shampoo.
> 3. Use the "nit comb" daily to remove the egg sacs that attach to the hair shafts.
> 4. Wash everyone's bedding, as well as all of your child's clothing.
> 5. Vacuum all of the furniture in the family room, living room, and bedrooms.
> 6. Put items that you can't wash into a sealed plastic bag and leave them there for several weeks before reusing.
> Repeat the first three steps in 1 week. If lice remain, contact your physician for additional assistance.

Before you finish reading the list, your own head starts to feel itchy. The amount of work involved is daunting and the thought of creepy, crawly creatures in your hair is revolting.

No matter what you've heard, however, head lice are nowhere near as bad as their reputation suggests. Having head lice doesn't mean you or your child is dirty. Head lice don't come from dirty people. They're not a plague or an affliction, and they don't carry any diseases. But they are a nuisance in every sense of the word: They can disrupt your household schedule and cause a lot of work for you.

Head lice are parasites that infest millions of people every year in the United States. They're spread through direct contact with a person with lice and through contact with combs, brushes, hats, scarves, and other infested items of clothing. Head lice can't live for more than a day or two without their human host.

You can get rid of head lice in a number of ways, although some are better than others. For years, lindane and other highly chlorinated pesticides were contained in the shampoos used against head lice. While this was previously considered safe, health-care professionals are now concerned that the amount of the lindane that can be absorbed through the skin is significant. It is therefore prudent to minimize your child's exposure to these chemicals to avoid the possible long-term toxic effects of pesticides. (See Smart Solutions 29 30 32)

The problem of exposing your child to toxic pesticides such as lindane becomes even more troublesome if you have to repeat applications of the treatment. As pediatricians and health-care professionals, we strongly recommend that you choose the least-toxic method available to get rid of head lice.

"Nit-Picking"

Whoever invented this word for the laborious tasks involving an enormous amount of detail surely understood head lice. Removing nits from the hair is the best way—but also the most labor-intensive way—to stop the infestation. Each nit is an egg that will hatch into a new louse. If you remove all of the nits, the lice will disappear. This is the least-toxic method for removing lice and nits, and it is the *only* method that should be used for children under 2 years old.

To remove the nits, you'll need a good bright light, a magnifying glass, and a fine-tooth nit comb (you can buy a nit comb at your local drugstore). Comb through the hair, section by tiny section, and remove any nits you find. Put the nits on some toilet paper and flush the paper down the toilet.

Remove every nit from every family member. You may need to do this for several days in a row to make sure that you get all the nits. Remember, the advantage to this method is that you don't have to use any toxic chemicals. (In addition, bedding should be washed, and any items that can't be washed should be tightly bagged and sealed in plastic for several weeks.)

Olive Oil

Using olive oil to treat head lice has many advocates and has some limited scientific basis supporting the claims that it's effective. This method consists of applying olive oil to the head and wrapping the hair in plastic wrap, on the theory that the lice will die of suffocation. The head wrap must remain in place for several hours for the oil to work. Once you remove the wrap, you'll need to wash your child's hair and then remove the nits with a fine-tooth comb. Most advocates of this method also advise repeating this treatment for several days.

Researchers at the Harvard School of Public Health found that in laboratory studies of lice and nits treated with olive oil, the oil showed some effectiveness in killing lice. You may wish to try this method out before considering more toxic alternatives.

Least-Toxic Chemical Shampoos

Most over-the-counter shampoos designed to remove head lice contain permethrin or a pyrethrin-type pesticide. Although permethrin- and pyrethrin-based shampoos are effective in treating head lice, you might need to repeat using the shampoo and the fine-tooth comb to bring the problem under control. These chemicals are considered to have low toxicity, but may be endocrine disrupters (See 92), so we advocate using them only as a last resort.

66 SMART SOLUTION
Use lead- and asbestos-free crayons.

☆☆
Important

△
Easy

Within the past few years, crayons (particularly crayons made in China) have been recalled a number of times because of their lead content. Crayons with lead can pose a particular health hazard to young children, as they're often sticking the crayons—or their hands that have just held the crayons—in their mouths.

When a child puts a crayon with lead in it into her mouth, she may ingest lead from the crayon. (See 19 24 26 for more on lead poisoning.)

The possibility of asbestos in crayons is also another cause for concern. In the spring of 2000, there was a media blitz surrounding the possibility that asbestos was present in Crayola crayons. The manufacturer (Binney & Smith, Inc.) assured the public that asbestos was not present, yet independent testing found some asbestos-like mineral fibers in the crayons. The controversy rests with the definition of asbestos: Although many mineral fibers share the same potential for the health effects attributed to asbestos, only those fibers that are actually used in a product that combats fire can be called "asbestos." In fact, the asbestos-like fibers found in some crayons cause the same health problems as asbestos and should be removed from crayons. (Binney & Smith has stated that it will remove any asbestos-like fibers from its crayons.)

The danger of asbestos is most serious if asbestos fibers are inhaled, beginning a cycle of lung scarring that can ultimately lead to asbestos-related diseases, such as lung cancer, much later in life. The ingestion of asbestos fibers has also been linked with cancer of the intestinal tract.

If you're concerned that your child may have been using crayons that had lead or asbestos in them, you don't need to panic. On your next routine visit to the pediatrician, tell him you'd like to have your child tested for lead poisoning. (It's an easy screening procedure that's recommended as part of routine pediatric care for children who may have had some exposure to lead.) And when you buy your child's next box of crayons, be sure to purchase a brand that is certified free of lead and asbestos. (The *Seattle Post-Ingelligencer* published such a list in 2000; you can find it at www.seattlep-i.com.)

As far as the asbestos goes, the likelihood that your child could have inhaled enough asbestos to cause health problems in later life from just using crayons is very small. In fact, there aren't even any blood or screening tests that would be helpful at this time, so the best thing you can do is make sure your child uses asbestos-free crayons in the future—and then not worry about it.

Keep in mind that a brief exposure to crayons that have asbestos-like materials or to crayons that have lead in them is a minimal risk to your child's health, but one that you want to avoid if you can. With asbestos, the risk of disease is also related to other lifestyle risks—for example, someone who smokes is 50 times as likely to develop lung cancer from an asbestos exposure than someone who doesn't smoke. With lead, the child's danger of lead poisoning is dependent upon his total ingestion of lead from a number of different sources. To protect your child from lead poisoning, eliminate every one of the lead sources that you can.

67
Find out about pesticide usage.

As we explained earlier in this book (see Smart Solutions 29–34), pesticides contain all sorts of toxic chemicals that may be harmful to children. For that reason, kids shouldn't be exposed to pesticides at all.

☆☆☆
Very Important

△
Easy

To make sure that your child isn't being exposed to pesticides at day care, encourage the day care not to routinely apply pesticides as a preventative. Instead, ask them to treat only known problems and to use exterminators that utilize Integrated Pest Management (IPM) techniques. You should also offer to call the local cooperative extension to learn how to control pests without using pesticides. (See 70)

As important as it is for the actual day care facility to not use pesticides, it's just as important that no one in the neighborhood spray pesticides near the day care without advance warning. (See 33) Some states, including New York and California, have enacted "neighbor notification" laws for pesticide spraying; this is a good project for a community group. (See 81) With advance warning, staff members can close the windows and bring in the toys—as well as make sure all the children stay inside the building.

68
Check the play area for toxic materials.

Of course you expect an outdoor play area to have swings, sliding boards, sandboxes, jungle gyms, and the like. What you shouldn't expect to see, however, are cans of weed killer, pesticides, spray paint, turpentine, and cleaning materials. Toxic products such as those should either not be used at all, or at the very least be locked away in an area that's not accessible to children.

☆☆☆
Very Important

△
Easy

69
Replace pressure-treated wood products.

Pressure-treated wood is often used in building playground equipment, decks, and picnic tables. As we mentioned in Smart Solution 44, the draw of using such lumber is that it stands up to the elements better and lasts longer than lumber that hasn't been treated. However, this type of wood is treated with toxic chemicals, specifically chromated copper arsenate (arsenic).

☆☆
Important

△
Easy

The concern here is that these toxic chemicals may leach out from the wood. One study, reported in the *Bulletin of Environmental Contamination and Toxicology* in 1997, showed that elevated levels of copper, chromium, and arsenic were found in soil beneath decks made of pressure-treated wood. Since children play in yards around decks, a child playing on the ground around the deck could ingest soil with these toxins in it if he puts his fingers in his mouth.

This is a potential hazard because arsenic is dangerous when ingested. Even if the levels of toxins in the soil are well below levels required for acute poisoning, such levels may still cause health problems.

The Consumer Product Safety Commission has not yet recommended that use of pressure-treated wood in consumer products be discontinued, but its tests have shown that arsenic can contaminate skin when the treated wood is handled. And that means that whenever your child plays on a treated wood playset or sits on a treated wood picnic table, any bare skin that comes in contact with the wood may be absorbing toxic chemicals.

Given the potential hazards of pressure-treated wood, we strongly recommend that you keep your children away from it. We suggest that the pressure-treated wood product be replaced with a nontoxic alternative. Untreated wood, especially untreated cedar, is a good choice.

If it's not possible to remove and replace the pressure-treated wood that your children have access to, consider coating the wood with paint or varnish to minimize the chance that arsenic will leach from the wood.

70 SMART SOLUTION
Prevent bug bites safely.

Insect bites are an almost unavoidable part of childhood and growing up. You may still remember your first bee sting, or the itch of multiple mosquito bites after those summer picnics.

Important

Most likely, your child gets lots of outdoor playtime at day care—and that means she's fair game for bug bites. So how can you protect her sensitive skin from being nibbled on?

Easy

For starters, dressing her in long-sleeved shirts and long pants (when the weather permits) tucked into socks helps minimize the amount of skin that's exposed. Washing her with unscented soaps and shampoos also helps to avoid attracting biting insects.

Beyond that, you may want to consider the judicious use of insect repellents if you know your child is going to be outdoors for a while in an insect-prone area, or in areas where mosquitoes or other insects carry disease.

The most effective repellents for thwarting mosquitoes and some other insects contain DEET (n,n diethyl toluamide). However, these products are also known to cause adverse effects. Rare reports of neurological problems and seizures associated with the use of DEET in children have been cited in medical literature. Although very uncommon, these potential health effects can be minimized by either not using DEET at all or using it sparingly.

The American Academy of Pediatrics recommends that if you must use DEET, you use a product containing no more than 10 percent DEET for children under 5 years old. Do not use DEET-containing products on infants. Use any products containing DEET only on your child's clothing—not on her skin. Make sure to avoid using it near her eyes and mouth, as well. And before using products containing DEET on your child, consult your own pediatrician or health-care provider.

Some nontoxic insect repellents have been advertised as effective in preventing mosquito bites. These include Avon Skin-So-Soft, certain preparations of herbs and garlic, and citronella oil. Although there's little scientific evidence that these products are effective, many people swear by them.

UNWELCOME GUESTS

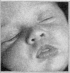

ONE OF the best ways to battle outdoor insect pests on your home turf is to learn about what a particular insect likes, and then do what you can to pull the welcome mat out from under it—or else stay indoors when it's outside. Here are some examples.

• Many mosquitoes prefer to feed from dusk until dawn; plan outdoor activities with that in mind. Eliminate standing water to make your yard less hospitable to them.

• Ticks like moist environments at the edges of lawns and wooded areas; keep lawns mowed on a regular basis to discourage ticks from taking up residence.

• Many ants and wasps are attracted to foods and fruity, sugary drinks. To be safe, drink sodas or fruit juices out of covered mugs.

If you're not sure about a particular pest's habits, call your local cooperative extension service for information.

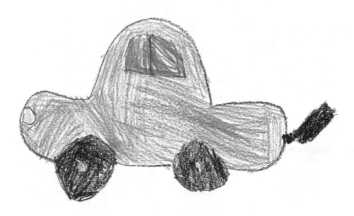

10 Ways to Make Your Child's School Safer

WHEN YOU send your child off to school each day, your primary concern should be the quality of the education he's receiving. Yet what's the point of a good education if your child is being exposed to toxic hazards that may impair his ability to learn or harm his health in the future?

After all, the chance of your child being exposed to toxic materials is just as great at school as it is anyplace else. And since he spends so much time at school, making sure his environment there is chemical-free is extremely important. Here are some steps to help you ensure that your child's learning environment is safe.

71 SMART SOLUTION
Be a school watchdog.

Starting or joining a group to review school environmental issues is a great way to solve current problems as well as prevent future ones. Your first step in becoming a school watchdog is to talk with the school administration or other parents in the school to find out if such a group already exists. If your school has a Parent Teacher Organization (PTO) or a Parent Teacher Association (PTA), perhaps that group will know what has been done in the past to review potential environmental problems in your school. They may even have an environment committee.

☆☆☆
Very
Important

△△
Moderately
Easy

If there is a group established already, offer to join them. Suggest that you would be willing to work with other parents to review environmental issues around the school. If no such group exists, think about bringing together a small group of parents and community residents to explore the issues. You may have already met some allies during talks with school officials or parents. Once you've formed a group, you can start looking at your concerns. Here's a format you can use as a guideline for solving problems.

Identify an easy issue to tackle. Tackling issues is like picking apples: Pick the low-hanging fruit first. An easy success is the best way to motivate a group to take further action and set more difficult goals. You may already know of an easily solved environmental problem at the school. Perhaps, for example, you've observed that the school buses park under the window of the first-grade classroom and idle their engines for 5 or 10 minutes every day before classes are released. Obviously, inhaling the fumes isn't good for the children, and you've noticed another area where the school could park the buses. That's an example of an easily solved environmental problem that a newly formed group can tackle.

Communicate through the right channels. Knowing the channels of communication in your school can go a long way in helping to bring an issue to the table. Does the school principal or a representative attend the PTO meetings? If so, that's a good place to make your committee's

MAKING IT HAPPEN

 WHEN TRYING to change a situation at school, make sure to utilize the expertise and connections of your committee members. For example, perhaps someone is a good writer and can make your case in the local newspaper. Maybe another member is well versed in how the school system contracts work.

Also keep your committee interested and on target. Make sure meetings are short and to the point (and come complete with refreshments!) and that everyone knows what's being done and who is doing it.

Talk about the successes of the group and praise the people making progress. Don't let roadblocks stop the group. Discuss problem areas as soon as you identify them and use the committee to come up with strategies to overcome them. Give credit, reassurance, and support to the people working on the projects that are running into problems, and reassess your strategy if you need to.

concerns known. Are there some teachers or a teachers' group who are interested in environmental issues? Does the PTO issue a regular report to the school administration? If so, that's a great way to communicate the concerns of your environmental committee as well as offer your solutions.

Present your case as a "win-win" situation for the children and for the school administration. Back up your arguments with some references. Is there an environmental expert in your community that you have convinced to become part of your committee? Perhaps this person could speak at the meeting where your concerns and possible solutions are discussed. If not, do you have authoritative material you can cite to back up your concerns?

Follow up to make sure the problem has been solved. Give the school administration a reasonable amount of time to ponder your solution and get the problem solved. If nothing happens, send a gentle reminder. School administrators and teachers are often overworked and underpaid. So give them the benefit of the doubt when things don't seem to be happening as fast as you'd like.

Choose your battles. If you propose 15 things that would be beneficial to the environmental health of the children at school and the school administration has already accomplished 9 of them, you have evidence of their good-faith efforts. So don't start World War III to get a minor issue resolved to your satisfaction if the administration hasn't yet dealt with it.

Solving More Difficult Issues

If you're having trouble reaching a resolution on an important issue, don't give up. Gather as much research as you can that supports your argument and makes sure you're on the right track. (You don't want to learn months down the road that a new law already solved your problem or that the premise that you're working on is wrong.) By doing this research, you can better formulate what arguments support your premise.

You should also strategize. Make a list of the people who support your position and note any key decision makers. Then determine who has the decision-making ability to solve your problem. In the idling school bus issue (assuming it is far more complicated than it originally appeared), perhaps the school principal has the authority to solve the problem. Or maybe the school superintendent sets the policy on school buses and negotiates the contracts with the bus companies each year.

Your next step is to develop a plan for convincing the decision maker to see things your way. In very complicated issues, this might involve a whole cascade of activities.

When all is said and done and the issue has been resolved, don't forget the kudos. After all, success has many parents. Thank every one of them, individually and in a group—more than once. Extol their talents. Don't forget your hard-working committee members, the forward-thinking superintendent of schools, or the principal that was convinced of the urgency of the particular issue.

72 SMART SOLUTION
Promote a smoke-free school.

Many school districts already have smoke-free schools. If yours doesn't, make this the top priority of your environmental committee. (See Smart Solution [71])

☆☆☆☆
Very
Important

However, even in smoke-free school systems, one big exception often exists: the teachers' lounge. Too often the teachers' lounge is a smoke-filled haven for smoking teachers who are taking a few minutes' respite from class. The thing to be concerned about here is your child's exposure to secondhand smoke. (See [15]) Unless the teachers' lounge has a totally separate air intake and exhaust system (not a likely situation in schools with central heating and the ordinary configuration of ventilation systems), the smoke from the teachers' lounge circulates throughout the school and becomes a part of your child's classroom and lungs.

△△
Moderately
Easy

The other area where your child can breathe in tobacco smoke is outside. When tobacco is prohibited indoors, smokers often congregate in a sheltered area right outside the school to smoke. When this area is directly under a classroom window or near the air intake vents for the school, the prohibited tobacco smoke has a free ride into the school and into your child's lungs.

What Can You Do?

Bring up the issue through the PTO to the school administration and ask them to remedy the problem. Also call your local health department and see if there are any regulations that will help with this situation. Put together a group of like-minded parents and join one of the antitobacco advocacy groups in your area, particularly one that's trying to pass legislation to address concerns such as these.

73 SMART SOLUTION
Promote Integrated Pest Management (IPM).

☆☆☆
Very
Important

△△
Moderately
Easy

Schools—with their cafeterias and lunches stored in lockers—provide an ideal indoor habitat for pests. According to cooperative extension services, common critters that inhabit school buildings include cockroaches, rodents, bees and wasps, ants, flies, and birds.

However, just because some schools may have pests in them doesn't mean your children need to be exposed to the quantity of pesticides that are currently used in schools. A recent survey by Connecticut environmental researchers showed that schools in 13 of the 16 school districts in Connecticut were treated with pesticides on a monthly basis, even though they may not have needed it. Surveys in other states have similarly shown that 85 to 90 percent of school districts routinely apply pesticides, whether or not there is evidence of need. Pesticides used indoors included bendiocarb, chlorpyrifos, cyfluthrin, cypermethrin, pyrethrin, piperonyl butoxide, tralomethrin, and bromadiolone. Many of these are toxic materials to which no child should be exposed.

In addition, seven school districts in Connecticut reported that townships were responsible for maintaining the athletic fields used by the schools; of these, 53 percent used herbicides, some of the more dangerous chemicals known. A total of 535,347 children in Connecticut were exposed to herbicides on soccer, football, and baseball playing fields.

The good news is that the control of any of the pests in your school does *not* require heavy, preventive sprayings of toxic pesticides that can be harmful to your child. The approach to pest management that gets the nod of approval from environmentalists and public health professionals is called Integrated Pest Management (IPM). This concept calls for an integrated approach to controlling pests—an approach that relies on a thorough knowledge of each pest and a nontoxic or least-toxic method of keeping the pest under control. In IPM, chemical pesticides are used only as the strategy of last resort.

We highly recommend that a school district considering IPM contact its local cooperative extension program to see if they have IPM advice for pests in the district's region.

Controlling Pests the IPM Way

The best, least-toxic way to control pests is to prevent them from ever infesting an area in the first place—make sure they can't get in, deny them access to food and water, and make the building uninhabitable.

In order to keep pests out, pest-management staff must learn everything they can about the pests in order to determine the best strategies to thwart them. This is the philosophy that needs to drive the pest-management staff that controls the pests in your child's school.

Don't hesitate to find out what the pest management professionals at your child's school know about a few common pests and how they plan to keep them under control. Don't be satisfied with an assurance that whatever the pesticide company is going to use "won't hurt anyone." (See Smart Solution [67])

The following tips are good examples of what we mean by controlling pests using IPM. Most of the following tips for controlling cockroaches are based on the pamphlet "Least Toxic Control of Pests in the Home and Garden" by the National Coalition against the Misuse of Pesticides.

To prevent cockroaches using IPM, you need to have a good understanding of the cockroach's habits—specifically, what it likes to eat and where it likes to live. Cockroaches will eat almost anything, including paper, cardboard, glue, and food scraps. They also need water to survive, which is why you'll often find them in bathrooms, kitchens, and areas with leaky pipes. Cockroaches are nocturnal bugs that hide in cracks and crevices during the day and retreat to them when threatened at night.

The IPM approach to cockroach control begins with eliminating the things that are attractive to them.

- Take away their water sources. Repair leaky pipes and faucets, and treat areas that have condensation on them.

- Wipe out their travel plans by repairing cracks and crevices with caulk or coating crevices with boric acid. (Boric acid poisons cockroaches. However, as with all pesticides, use with caution and keep it away from children.)

- Make sure cockroaches don't have a free meal. Thoroughly clean countertops and cooking surfaces and make sure they are crumb-free.

These are only a few of the nontoxic methods available for getting rid of cockroaches. For more information on controlling pests such as cockroaches through IPM, see "Resources" on page 145.

SMART SOLUTION

74 Find out if your school has had lead or asbestos problems in the past.

This is a great project for the parent group that's working on environmental issues. (See Smart Solution 71) The first place to start may be the PTO (Parent Teacher Organization), the principal, or the school custodian. Here are some questions you'll want to know the answers to.

☆☆☆
Very
Important

△△
Moderately
Easy

- Has the school been painted recently? If so:

  Who did it?

  Was the outside of the school sandblasted?

  Did anyone check to see if there was lead paint on the outside of the school before sandblasting was done?

- Have renovations been done to the school's interior? If so:

  Was the contractor a certified lead paint contractor?

  Was there old lead paint in the school?

- Has any of the school been demolished to make way for new construction? If so:

  Who did it? Did they find any asbestos or lead paint in the building?

  How was the rest of the school protected from the dust from the demolition?

- How old is the school? (Schools built before 1970 are more likely to contain lead paint and asbestos insulation than schools built after that date.)

- Has there been any construction recently in the school?

- How has the school's boiler or furnace been working?

- Has a new furnace been installed? If so:

  How recently was the new furnace installed?

  What happened to the old furnace?

  Was there asbestos covering the old furnace?

  Was there asbestos found on the heating pipes that carry heat to the other parts of the buildings?

Once you find out the answers, use them to determine whether the problem is severe, as well as help you make your case for eradicating the problem. This way, you'll have a good point of reference to work from when determining the severity of lead or asbestos problems.

Lead Paint in Schools

If you've been reading this book in sequential order, you know by now how serious the threat of lead poisoning is to your child's health. (See Smart Solutions ⟨19⟩–⟨28⟩ for a thorough discussion of lead paint.) Chipping, peeling, and flaking lead paint is an especially serious health hazard for children under the age of 6 years. If your school has a nursery, kindergarten, or day care, these are the most vulnerable areas—and the ones you want to focus on in your discussions of lead paint in the schools. If these classrooms haven't already been checked for lead paint, they definitely should be. If lead paint is present, call your local or state health department to find out what steps need to be taken to insure that the children are not at risk for lead poisoning.

Another potentially serious source of lead poisoning in schools is caused by untrained workers who sandblast lead paint on the outside of the school building (see ⟨91⟩) or an adjacent building, or who use a propane torch to remove old lead paint from interior or exterior trim (see ⟨21⟩). Sandblasting lead paint can create a lot of airborne lead dust and also can result in accumulation of leaded debris inside and outside the school. Torching lead paint can create highly toxic lead fumes that children, teachers, and workers can inhale.

If you discover that workers have sandblasted lead paint at your school or an adjacent building or that uncertified contractors have done renovations in areas where lead paint is present, contact your local or state health department for guidance on what you need to do. You may need to have the dust in the school tested to determine whether elevated lead levels are present. If there are, your next step is to call in certified lead paint removal contractors for a professional cleanup so that the school will be safe for your children.

About Asbestos

Asbestos is an umbrella term for a group of six naturally occurring fibrous minerals. Asbestos mines in Canada, Russia, and South Africa yield rocks that contain these thin, nearly indestructible fibers that resist heat, acid, and fire. Since the 1920s, billions of tons of asbestos have been used in homes, schools, and public buildings. The heaviest use of asbestos occurred in buildings built in the 1950s and 1960s. In the 1970s, the use of asbestos rapidly declined as the health hazards of asbestos became better known. Such hazards include lung cancer and malignant mesothelioma (a cancer of the chest and abdomen lining). These cancers can occur years after inhaling asbestos fibers: Lung cancer can occur 10 to 30 years after exposure to asbestos fibers, while mesothelioma generally occurs 20 to 50 years after exposure. All new use of asbestos in all forms is banned in the United States.

If you suspect your school has asbestos in it, arrange to have a certified inspector perform a visual inspection. He can then examine pieces of suspect material under an electron microscope to determine whether the material is really asbestos. Do not have an inspector take an air sample. Air sampling identifies only those asbestos particles that are airborne at a single moment in time, and asbestos is released into the air intermittently, such as when a hot-air heating system comes on and blows particles throughout the building.

Should Asbestos Always Be Removed?

Although the hazards of asbestos and the danger of improper asbestos removal were known by the 1970s, there was an incident some 20 years later in the schools of New York City in the early 1990s. By that time the federal Asbestos Hazard Emergency Response Act (AHERA) law was in place (see "Legal Protection" on page 106) and schools were inspecting and removing asbestos as required by AHERA. Unfortunately, in New York City, unqualified asbestos contractors were hired to do asbestos removal and instead created asbestos contamination in various schools throughout the city.

Parental concerns reached a fever pitch. A debate raged over what should be done, and the opening of schools was delayed in September.

As a result of the very public debate over the New York City schools' asbestos problem, health and municipal officials developed some guidelines about when asbestos should be removed from buildings and when it's safer to encapsulate it and leave it in place. Here are the guidelines.

- If asbestos is in poor condition, with apparent flaking and friability, it needs to be removed by a licensed, certified asbestos removal expert.

- If the asbestos is in good condition, with no flaking or cracking, it's better to leave well enough alone, consider putting physical barriers between it and children, and continue to monitor its condition on a regular basis.

ALL ASBESTOS IS DANGEROUS

 SIX DIFFERENT types of fibrous minerals are classified as "asbestos" when they're used for fire-retardant purposes. However, the asbestos industry and its consultants have mounted an extensive and highly misleading campaign in an attempt to persuade consumers that some forms of asbestos can be used safely. Like their counterparts in the tobacco industry, the industry sees benefit in denying the health dangers of their product. The argument they use is that different types of asbestos vary in their hazards and that the most widely used type of asbestos (Canadian crysotile asbestos) has minimal risks. This simply isn't true. All types of asbestos present health hazards, as they are all composed of tiny, nearly indestructible fibers that can be inhaled and that then lodge themselves in the lung tissue and cause irritation, scarring, and sometimes cancer.

What Do I Do about Asbestos Exposure?

If your child has already been exposed to asbestos, don't panic. He doesn't need to have any sort of medical screening because asbestos exposure doesn't produce any detectable physical damage until an average of 20 to 50 years after exposure. In particular, don't get a chest x-ray: It will reveal nothing in regard to the asbestos and will only expose your child to unnecessary radiation. Instead of worrying, use all your parental insights, guidance, and teaching to make sure your child does not become a smoker. People exposed to asbestos and who take up smoking are 50 times more likely to develop asbestos-related lung cancer than those people exposed to asbestos who don't smoke.

So don't wait until your child is a teenager to talk about smoking. These days, smoking is a childhood disease. According to national statistics, the vast majority of adult smokers began smoking in their childhood or teens. Few adults take up the smoking habit.

What Can Parent Groups Do?

You can make sure that the legally mandated inspections under AHERA were done in your child's school. Under federal law, parents have the right to request and examine school records. If the school administration doesn't respond to a written request for records, report it to the nearest Environmental Protection Agency (EPA) regional office.

LEGAL PROTECTION

THE 1984 Asbestos Hazard Emergency Response Act (AHERA) was passed to protect children and school employees from the hazards of asbestos in schools. Federal funds were made available to financially needy schools for investigation and remediation.

Under AHERA, schools are required to systematically inspect every room and every surface for the presence of asbestos every 3 years. The inspections must be done by properly qualified, professional inspectors and contractors, and parents and teachers must be informed of the inspections.

Make sure that proper asbestos abatement was done if asbestos was found. A review of school records should show whether a properly trained asbestos contractor did the work.

An asbestos problem taken care of by certified asbestos abatement contractors should leave you with nothing to worry about. If, instead, inexperienced and uncertified contractors did the abatement, contact the EPA and your local or state health department for guidance on what to do next.

75 SMART SOLUTION
Make sure the drinking water is lead-free.

In many older schools, you'll find that the drinking water is contaminated by lead because some older schools, like older homes, have lead pipes in their plumbing. They may also have lead solder in their plumbing (lead solder was banned from use by the federal government in 1986). When water sits in these lead pipes overnight, over a weekend, or during school vacations, it's possible for a small quantity of the lead from the plumbing system to leach into the drinking water. (This is particularly likely to happen in areas where the water is acidic.) Lead has also been found in some types of water fountains. When children drink the water, they will also ingest the lead that is present in the water. Since childhood lead poisoning results from a child's cumulative exposure to lead from many sources in the environment—such as ingesting lead paint chips and dust along with lead in drinking water—it's important to eliminate lead from every possible source in the environment.

☆☆
Important

Easy

The Environmental Protection Agency (EPA) shares your concern over lead in the drinking water in schools and has published guidelines for schools to prevent lead poisoning. (See "Resources" on page 145 for more information). Under these guidelines, schools are required to test their water in a prescribed fashion and in accordance with EPA guidelines. If lead is detected in the water, the source must be identified and the problem fixed.

SMART SOLUTION

76 Take a stroll outside the school.

Armed with "An Environmental Checklist for Your Neighborhood" on page 79, take a leisurely walk around the school's neighborhood to look for potential environmental hazards. (This is a great activity for a newly formed environmental group—see Smart Solution [71].) Keep your eyes open for the things listed below.

☆☆
Important

△
Easy

SITE OR ITEM	POTENTIAL HAZARDS
Gasoline station	Leaking fuel tanks underground; oil or gasoline spills into the soil; cleaning and degreasing fluid spills
Industrial site/factory (current or abandoned)	Industrial chemical spills or emissions; ground contamination at old industrial sites; school grounds contaminated by construction at the site
Outflow pipe	Toxic chemicals or sewage
Abandoned drums	Toxic chemicals
Discarded chemicals	Toxic chemicals
Landfill	Methane gas; toxic materials
Community compost site	Molds, allergens, and hazardous materials
Garbage transfer station	Hazardous materials
Construction or demolition site	Toxic materials; excessive dust; runoff of lead and other toxic materials into water
Discarded automobiles	Automobile fluids leaking into soil or water

When you've finished your field trip around the school's neighborhood, evaluate your list. The first thing you should do is break the problem areas into two separate groups.

Toxic materials that need immediate attention. Examples of these include abandoned drums with some contents, oil or gasoline spills in waterways, raw sewage spills, and discarded chemicals. If you find any of these situations, immediately call your local police, fire, or health department.

Potential hazards that need more investigation. Make a list of the potential hazards you've found, such as a construction site, ranking them in order of importance to the health of the school children. Decide which issues you're able to tackle now and which need additional research.

If you've identified a potential hazard but don't have the ability to address it right away, call it to the attention of a responsible agency anyway (and do it in writing). Some agencies you might consider: your child's school district, the local health department, or the municipal government.

Getting to Work

For the issue or issues you've identified as potential environmental hazards, decide what additional information you need to help you determine whether your group should go ahead and take on the issue.

For example, if you found a gasoline station or industrial site in your school's neighborhood, you'll want to investigate whether the groundwater, air, or soil is contaminated. Contact your local health department, give them the exact location of the site, and ask if there are any records of environmental hazards or regulatory actions at the site. Also check the EPA Toxic Release Inventory at www.scorecard.org or your state's department of the EPA to determine what's permitted to be released into the air. Research the potential health effects of any of the chemical releases permitted.

Once you've determined that you've found an environmental issue that your group wants to work on, see 71 for detailed information on how to tackle the problem.

77

SMART SOLUTION
Make sure science labs are safe.

New science and chemistry laboratories use far fewer toxic materials than older chemistry laboratories. And well-managed science experiments should pose no threat to a child's health. However, what may be sitting on a shelf in the old science lab storage closet can yield a frightening array of toxic and even explosive materials, some of which pose life-threatening hazards. Here are some materials that have been found in high school chemistry labs' old storage areas.

☆
Good
Idea

△
Easy

CHEMICAL	HAZARD
Benzene	A highly toxic solvent that can cause leukemia.
Carbon tetrachloride	A versatile and universal solvent once used in stamp collecting to bring out the water marks on the stamps. It's highly toxic to the liver and shouldn't be used without respiratory and skin protection.
Ether	Highly explosive. As ether ages, it can form explosive peroxides. Removal of old containers of ether requires a bomb squad.
Hexane	Acute inhalation exposure causes dizziness, giddiness, slight nausea, and headache. Chronic exposure causes nervous system dysfunction, numbness in the extremities, muscular weakness, blurred vision, headache, fatigue.
Old hydrochloric or sulfuric acid	Deteriorating acid containers can emit toxic fumes that can react with other lab chemicals. Can cause bone damage and burned lungs.
Old hydrofluoric acid	Hydrofluoric acid is a highly toxic substance that can eat through bone and etch glass. It shouldn't be used in high school laboratories. If hydrofluoric acid is in a deteriorating container, it poses a direct health threat to anyone who touches it.
Mercury	Mercury vaporizes readily at room temperature and is extremely toxic when inhaled or handled. It causes brain damage.
Picric acid	Aging picric acid can crystallize and can explode when jostled or even moved on the shelf. Removal requires a bomb squad.
Toluene	Toxic solvent; breathing high levels of toluene affects brain function and can cause central nervous system symptoms such as headaches, confusion, dizziness, sleepiness, and memory loss.

Given the number of chemicals out there that can cause serious problems in science class, you as a parent should:

- Ask the school administration for permission to review their protocol and procedures for maintenance of the high school chemistry storage room.

- Find out how old the school is and how long chemicals have been stored there.

- Determine when the storeroom was last surveyed for aging chemicals and by whom.

- Ask what teachers do to be sure they don't have old or unlabeled chemicals on their shelves.

- Find out if there are any other old storage areas where school chemicals are kept.

If your school doesn't have any sort of protocol for maintaining science lab chemicals, contact your local health department and ask whether they routinely inspect school laboratory storage rooms. If not, ask if they know who is responsible for doing so.

If no one is minding the store(room), bring this up as an issue of concern to your school administration, perhaps through the PTO. Ask them to have the school science lab storeroom evaluated by a qualified professional.

78 SMART SOLUTION
Review those art supplies.

Art supplies contain lots of toxic substances. See the opposite page for a list of art supplies and what toxic materials may be in them.

☆☆
Important

You're probably thinking, "How can I make sure all the art products in my child's school are safe to use?" Well, the good news is that in 1998, the federal government passed the Labeling of Hazardous Art Materials Act. Crayons, paint sets, chalk, modeling clay, colored pencils, and other art products must be labeled to show whether the materials contain the potential to pose a chronic hazard. If the materials are not toxic, the label will state "Conforms to ASTM D-4236."

△
Easy

A good project for the environmental committee (See Smart Solution [71]) or the PTO would be to review the art supplies used by your child's class and recommend that the least-toxic alternatives be used whenever possible. Here's a list of supplies and points you should keep in mind.

Oil paints. Oil paints aren't for young children. Only students who are old enough to avoid putting their hands or their paintbrushes in their mouths should use them. In more advanced art classes, the teacher should make sure budding young artists do not develop the habit of "tipping" their brushes (bringing the fine hairs of the brush together by putting the brush in the mouth). The beautiful colors of cadmium yellow, cobalt blue, and manganese purple contain some very toxic metals if ingested.

Art Supply	Toxin and Its Harmful Effects
Oil paints	*Lead:* impaired brain function, decreased IQ, coma, convulsion, death *Cadmium:* lung, kidney, and digestive tract damage *Cobalt:* respiratory irritation; rash *Manganese:* central nervous system disorders *Turpentine* (used in cleanup of oil paints): headache, dizziness, decreased central nervous system function; liver, kidney, and blood disorders
Pastels	*Pigment dusts:* lung and respiratory problems, impaired brain function, decreased IQ, convulsion *Cadmium:* lung, kidney, and digestive tract damage *Mercury compounds:* brain, kidney, and liver damage
Magic Markers	*Xylene:* headaches, dizziness, confusion, balance problems; breathing problems *Propyl alcohol:* headache, drowsiness, incoordination, nausea, vomiting, gastrointestinal distress *Methyl isobutyl ketone* (in Dry Erase markers used on whiteboards): eye irritant; headache, nausea, vomiting, incoordination, drowsiness
Rubber cement	*N-heptane:* respiratory tract irritation; lightheadedness, dizziness, muscle incoordination, nausea; abdominal pain; lung damage
Spray adhesives	*N-heptane, 1,1,1-trichloroethane:* dizziness, headache, nausea
Ceramics	*Clay dust* (silica): respiratory irritation *Lead:* impaired brain function, decreased IQ, convulsion *Cadmium:* lung, kidney, and digestive tract damage *Talc:* (See 7) *Asbestos-like materials:* respiratory distress and disease *Sulfur dioxide:* life-threatening bronchospasm in susceptible individuals *Carbon monoxide* (from the kiln firing): oxygen deprivation in red blood cells; death

When using solvents to clean brushes, students should use turpenoid, odorless paint thinner, or odorless mineral spirits rather than turpentine; and the classroom should also be adequately ventilated.

Pastels. Because imported pastels can contain toxic heavy metals such as lead, cadmium, and mercury compounds, students using them must be careful not to inhale them. These are not good art supplies for young children. Although oil pastels are not as dusty as chalk pastels, they still may contain toxic heavy metals if the pastels are imported. Use ASTM D-4236–approved chalk instead.

Magic Markers. Make sure the markers do not contain toxic solvents and are ASTM D-4236–approved. Avoid scented markers, which can encourage children to taste them.

Rubber cement. Rubber cement contains n-heptane, a solvent that can cause dizziness, headache, and blurring of consciousness at higher doses. Substitute water-based glue, such as white glue, or double-sided tape.

Spray adhesives. These products contain petroleum distillates and a variety of other chemicals, such as propane, acetone, and isopropyl alcohol. Exposure to these through inhalation can cause dizziness, headache, drowsiness, lack of coordination, nausea, and other symptoms. The aerosol can insures that the toxins will be dispersed into the air where a child can inhale them. In light of that, we think art students should avoid spray adhesives when possible. If spray adhesives are critical to a particular project, students should make sure to use them in a well-ventilated place (like outdoors) and with OSHA (Occupational Safety and Health Administration)-approved respiratory protection. Or they should choose CP/AP clear acrylic emulsions to fix their drawings. (CP/AP stands for Certified Product/Approved Product. To carry either of these seals, an authority on toxicology from the Art and Craft Materials Institute must have evaluated the product and determined that there aren't materials in sufficient quantity to be toxic or to injure the body even if ingested.)

Pottery and ceramics. Keep the dust down as best as possible and the children's hands out of their mouths when working with pottery and ceramics. Use only nontoxic, certified lead-free paints and glazes.

79 SMART SOLUTION
Have a hazardous spill plan.

Occasionally schools experience spills (such as oil or cleaning materials) that can be hazardous to your child's health. Many times these spills are not part of an emergency plan. Valuable time is wasted while someone waits for staff to try to find out what agency is responsible for helping them with the problem.

☆☆
Important

△△
Moderately
Easy

So check your school's protocol for the handling of spills. If they don't have one, offer to write one for them. Here are some potential spills you'll want covered in the protocol.

- Science lab accidents, including broken mercury thermometers

- Oil tank overfills or other petroleum spills

- Sewage spills or sewage malfunctions

- Cleaning agents

You'll also want to include protocols to follow for accidental mixing of cleaning agents (such as bleach and ammonia) that result in toxic emissions, and overapplication of pesticides in the classroom (See Smart Solutions 29 – 32).

A good protocol should list who is in charge, along with two backup contacts. The phone numbers (day, evening, and weekend) should be listed for all of the people in charge. These phone numbers should also be registered with the local police and fire departments.

The protocol should spell out in detail what has to happen, step by step, for any of the above situations—and any others that may be identified as potential problems in the area of your school (such as a chemical factory next door).

80 SMART SOLUTION
Do roofing repairs when school is over.

Roofing tars contain noxious and hazardous materials derived from petroleum products (polycyclic aromatic hydrocarbons). Research has shown that workers who use these roofing tars and pitches on a regular basis have as much as five times greater risk of lung cancer than the rest of the population.

☆☆
Important

△△
Moderately Easy

When roofing tars and pitches are heated, they emit noxious fumes that can cause eye and nose irritation, nausea, headaches, and malaise. That's why the ideal situation involves doing any roofing repairs when school's not in session. If roofing projects for your school must take place during the school season, recommend that the school administration assure that the contractors:

- Turn off air intakes in the vicinity while applying tars.

- Close windows on the side of the building where roofing vapors are present.

- Keep the pot of roofing tar away from the area where fumes will get into classrooms. They should also keep the pot covered except when they're using it.

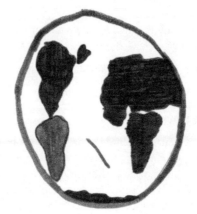

10 Tips for Avoiding Neighborhood Dangers

HOW OFTEN have you told your child, "Look both ways before crossing the street." "Don't touch stray dogs." "Wear that helmet when your ride your bike—and make sure you stay on the bike path."

Probably more times than you care to think about, right? Because every time your child leaves the shelter of your home to venture out into your neighborhood, you worry about his safety and hope that he makes it home in one piece.

But stray dogs and traffic aside, there may be other dangers in your neighborhood—dangers that could be quietly affecting your child's health. And no careful reminders from you can help protect him from things such as toxic chemicals released into the air from industries, pesticides sprayed on park grounds, herbicides sprayed on roadsides to control weeds, contaminated water, and lead paint on buildings.

Those examples are just some of the dangers that you need to be aware of. Don't feel as though your hands are tied, however, when it comes to eliminating such dangers in your neighborhood. Chances are, you're not the only one in town concerned about the effects of environmental hazards on your child's health. Once you gather community support, you'll be surprised and pleased at the changes you'll be able to set in motion.

81 SMART SOLUTION
Get involved with a community group.

Find out if a group exists in your community to address environmental issues. If one does, join them and see what sort of problems they've identified and what steps they've taken to address those problems. Add your own ideas and some of the ones suggested in this book.

☆☆
Important

△△
Moderately Easy

If a community group isn't already established, gather a few neighbors and get one going. Your group doesn't have to be huge; you can start out with four or five people and grow larger as the need arises.

Your first task should be surveying your neighborhood for environmental hazards. (See Smart Solution 82) Then develop your own checklist of problems you want to address. Don't be discouraged if the list of problems seems overwhelming—just tackle them one at a time instead of trying to solve everything at once.

Choose a few easy tasks first to get the group going and give them some easy "wins." For example, you may want to concentrate first on safety issues as opposed to toxic ones. Maybe you'd like to have a stop sign installed on a busy road where your children cross the street. Or maybe you'd like to see a fence installed around a hazardous storm drain next to the local park.

Once your group has some success under its belt, you can move on to bigger issues such as researching your water supply, checking on the toxic releases in your neighborhood, and pushing for Integrated Pest Management (IPM) techniques.

FOLLOW THE LEADER

WHEN YOUR community group decides it's ready to tackle a big project, you should establish a group leader (if you haven't already done so). Help the leader delegate tasks to others in the group and encourage the other members to work with the leader to keep things moving.

By establishing a leader and then breaking the big project into small tasks (that can be accomplished easily by busy people with lots on their minds!), your project will probably go much smoother, and you'll end up with a better and more satisfying result.

82

Conduct a neighborhood survey.

How well do you know the neighborhood you live in? Have you explored it with the eyes of a child? Do you know its hidden secrets?

☆☆
Important

As families move in and out of neighborhoods more frequently than in previous decades, many parents don't live in the neighborhood where they grew up. While moving to a new area can be an exciting adventure, there's also a disadvantage to not knowing your neighborhood well.

△△
Moderately Easy

Even families that stay closer to home may not know their neighborhoods as well as they think. As things change, communities age and the infrastructure becomes more fragile. Sewage pipes leak, wells become contaminated, new industry moves in. (See "Hidden Dangers" on the opposite page for three examples of large environmental problems.)

Even small problems can be large hazards. For example, open drainpipes that contain runoff from agricultural fields can look like great hiding places to your kids. Young explorers in the woods can unearth buried industrial waste. The terrain beyond the edge of your subdivision may look very different and present different environmental hazards than those in the manicured uniformity of your development. Areas where people dump things illegally can present problems ranging from broken glass to dangerous chemicals.

That's why the best way to be sure your children are protected from environmental dangers in your neighborhood is to conduct your own neighborhood survey. Gather a few like-minded neighbors together and divide up the work. Here are some of the things your group should tackle.

Check out the history of the land on which your neighborhood was built. Municipal or town records are a good place to start, as is your local health department or town historical society. Look for potentially dangerous environmental uses of the land in the past, such as former industrial facilities, town dumps, and manufacturing sites. Ask about the use of land as former farmland and about the agricultural use of pesticides. Check for hazardous waste sites in your community using the Agency for Toxic Substances and Disease Registry (ATSDR) at www.atsdr.cdc.gov.

Check the source of your drinking water. See Smart Solution 83 for an in-depth discussion of issues with your drinking water. Visit the EPA's Web site (www.epa.gov) for additional information on drinking water in your community.

HIDDEN DANGERS

 THERE MAY be hidden (or maybe even not so hidden) environmental dangers in your neighborhood. Some may be potentially deadly. Here are a few examples.

Woburn, Massachusetts, is a community that had a hidden environmental health threat. A neighborhood of under 50,000 people in the shadow of Boston, Woburn is an old community with a history of manufacturing and industrial activities. After World War II, Woburn became a suburb, and the new suburban houses in the area were served by two municipal wells. In 1979, the town learned that the wells had been contaminated from buried industrial waste containing myriad toxic chemicals including trichlorethylene, perchlorethylene, and arsenic. The wells were quickly closed, but the damage had already been done. That year, 12 children who lived in Woburn were diagnosed with childhood leukemia. Six of them had lived in homes served by the contaminated wells, and their mothers had consumed the contaminated water when pregnant. Although no guilt on anyone's part was proven in court, the community is still concerned over the threat of toxins and leukemia.

You've probably heard of Love Canal, New York, which had its hidden environmental secrets as well. A community on the edge of industrialized Buffalo, Love Canal became the nation's largest hazardous waste site in the nation in the mid-1970s. Occidental Petroleum admitted to dumping tens of thousands of tons of hazardous chemicals into Love Canal, contaminating the community's soil and water. The whole community became a wasteland as residents moved out without being able to sell their homes because of the contamination. For over 15 years, the community was a ghost town. Today, slowly, some parts of the community are being reinhabited.

Times Beach, Missouri, experienced an environmental disaster of its own that could have been prevented. Crisscrossed with dusty unpaved roads, Times Beach became contaminated with PCBs (polychlorinated biphenyls) when a local contractor spread PCB-contaminated oil on the roads to keep down the dust. PCBs and dioxins, a by-product of heating PCBs, are potentially cancer-causing chemicals. They also can damage the developing brain and cause learning disabilities and behavioral problems. The community was evacuated by federal authorities and remained uninhabitable for many years.

These environmental problems were all potentially preventable before catastrophe struck. In Woburn, municipal well-water testing might have found the problem before children died. In Love Canal, the dumping of huge quantities of hazardous waste could have been discovered and stopped before the community was damaged, and intelligent city planning could have prevented the building of homes and schools on this massive waste site. And in Times Beach, the use of waste oil (that should have been tested before its use) to keep the dust down was risky business; the contamination of that oil with PCBs was an accident waiting to happen.

Take a bird's-eye view of your neighborhood and the surrounding area. Start with some good maps of your community. A topographical map shows the hills, valleys, rivers, and streams. (You can order topographic maps from the United States Geological Survey for about $4, plus shipping and handling. Their Internet address is http://search.usgs.gov.) A detailed local road map is also useful, as is a good road map of up to 100 miles or so of your area. Using the maps, look for potential trouble spots.

- Industrial areas that may discharge waste products into rivers or streams that flow through your community

- Farmland whose pesticides may flow into rivers

- Sewage treatment plants that may release sewage into a river or estuary

- Power plants that may pose a threat from nuclear power accidents or from toxic emissions from their stacks

- Airports and transportation centers that may use toxic chemicals to keep the buses, trains, or planes operating

Walk around your neighborhood and look at it from your child's point of view. Your child can find adventure in many things you may not even give a second thought to, such as abandoned industrial lots and discarded containers filled with strange-looking liquids. But these items can be hazardous to your child's health. So find out where they are and keep your child away from them.

Once you've completely surveyed your neighborhood and have developed your list of problem areas, see 81.

83

SMART SOLUTION
Find out where your water comes from.

Just because your water tastes okay doesn't mean it's not contaminated. That's why it's important to know where you water comes from—and what's in it. If your drinking water comes from a well (see "Drinking Water Defined" on the opposite page for a definition of well water), here are some things you need to know.

Who assures its quality? If your municipality owns the well, ask whether the municipality conducts regular tests of the water quality. If the well is on your property, then the upkeep of water quality is your responsibility.

☆☆
Important

△
Easy

DRINKING WATER DEFINED

HERE ARE a few terms to help you understand what we're talking about in the discussion of drinking water.

Well water. Underground water brought to the surface by pumping through pipes.

Aquifer. An underground water source, typically consisting of permeable rock where groundwater has accumulated over time.

Groundwater. Water contained in aquifers below the earth's surface. Groundwater is replenished over time as rain and snow percolate into the ground.

Watershed. All of the land whose rain and snow contribute to the groundwater you drink.

How often is the water tested? For municipally owned wells, a law dictates the schedule. (Ask for the testing schedule so you'll know how often it's done.) For your own well, you should hire someone to test the water annually. If you have a contractor that does routine maintenance on your well, ask if he knows a lab that will test the water. (Make sure the lab has the appropriate certification from the state to do well water testing and that the sample is collected as directed by the lab.) Or ask your local health department for the names of certified laboratories for the testing of well water.

What's been found in the well water in the past? If volatile organic chemicals—such as those that signal a potential petroleum or gasoline spill—appear in the well water, it's important to frequently monitor the water. State and local health officials should also be notified of the problem so they can help remediate the situation.

If coliform bacteria (*E. coli*) have been found in the well, the well may need to be disinfected. Again, state and local health officials should be notified so they can help fix the problem.

Are there contaminated aquifers in your area? Aquifers are the rocky environments your water flows through. To find out if any are contaminated, contact your state or local health department. Use the Freedom of Information Law to request records of any aquifer contamination from local, state, and federal officials.

Have any of the features you discovered in Smart Solution 82 **impacted your well water?** Consider the potential implications of what you found in your neighborhood environmental survey. Most farms and golf courses use large amounts of pesticides and fertilizers that leach into the groundwater. Transportation facilities use petroleum products that have been linked to contamination of groundwater in some areas.

What's the geology of your area like? Some geological formations or conditions can be problematic for well water.

Some communities are built primarily on fractured bedrock, a geological rock formation that is filled with cracks and crevices. With fractured bedrock, wells can become contaminated in an unpredictable manner from a site very far away from the well. For example, gasoline leaking into fractured bedrock from a gasoline station that's miles away from your home can end up in your well water by traveling along a series of cracks in the bedrock.

Sandy soil and a high water table are common features in low-lying coastal areas; they combine to allow contaminants to reach well water very easily. Areas of Long Island, New York, and Cape Cod, Massachusetts, have this type of geological foundation. In both areas, gasoline and other fuel leaks have contaminated portions of the aquifer.

If your drinking (well) water comes from groundwater (either directly from a river or from a manmade reservoir) you need to know the answers to these questions.

How is your water tested? Who does the testing? What have they found?

How is the watershed area protected? If your watershed area (see "Drinking Water Defined" on page 119) includes large tracts of farmland where excessive amounts of pesticides and fertilizers are used, you'll want to know if any of these appear in your drinking water. Ask your water supplier if they test for pesticide and fertilizer contamination and find out the results.

If your watershed area includes large cattle or dairy farms, ask your water supplier how your water is protected against parasites such as cryptosporidium, which is carried by infected cattle. Microscopic cryptosporidium cysts can get into the water supply and cause diarrhea and more severe complications in people with damaged immune systems. In 1993 in Milwaukee, for example, there was a massive cryptosporidium outbreak, which was linked to the municipal water treatment plant. Cryptosporidium (probably from animal farms in the vicinity) washed into the streams and rivers in spring rains and passed through the treatment plants' filtration system without being removed—and then into the drinking water. The "malfunction" was the inability of the filtration system to remove the contaminants necessary to produce safe drinking water. The best way to prevent the problem is not to let cattle graze in sensitive watershed areas. Some filtration systems are thought to be useful in limiting the numbers of cysts in the water supply, but are not as effective as keeping the cows out.

Does your community use river water? River water can be problematic if the river is used as a dumping ground upstream or if the river receives agricultural runoff. And that very well may be the case because industries and farms are allowed by law to discharge certain quantities of chemical by-products into the air and water. If the river is located downstream of industries or is surrounded by farms, you may want to think twice about what's in your water.

84

SMART SOLUTION

Find out what chemicals are being released into your air and water.

By law, industrial facilities and manufacturers are permitted to release certain amounts of chemical by-products into the air and water of the surrounding community. Supposedly the health impact of such releases is minimized by the fact that only by-product amounts that are aren't known to cause health problems are allowed to be released.

☆☆
Important

△
Easy

The theory behind this law is that "dilution is the solution to pollution." When small quantities of materials are released into large quantities of air or water, they dissipate quickly. However, this theory isn't all it's cracked up to be. When chemical by-products are released into an increasingly congested and residential community, unanticipated health effects may occur. And often there is not just one but many polluting facilities nearby. A chemical soup can form in the air or water. And who can be sure that that the levels of contaminants in the air or water are always safe, especially for small children?

The Environmental Protection Agency (EPA) maintains a list of permitted chemical releases in your community. You can find out about those releases by consulting the EPA's Toxic Release Inventory at www.scorecard.org. Under the Community Right-to-Know Act, you have a right to know what sorts of chemicals industrial sources are releasing into the air and water of your community.

85 SMART SOLUTION
Push for IPM techniques.

Pest management doesn't have to mean the excessive use of pesticides. These days, communities all across the country are adopting safer means of controlling insects, rodents, and other pests. In fact, some communities are adopting "sunset ordinances"—local legislation that declares the community's intent to eliminate the use of pesticides on their property by a given date.

☆☆☆
Very Important

△△
Moderately Easy

Integrated Pest Management (IPM) is a relatively new technique for dealing with pests using the least-toxic alternatives available. IPM requires a major shift in thinking. Instead of laying down a chemical barrier to eliminate pests, proponents of IPM manage pests instead to keep them from becoming a health or environmental threat. (See Smart Solution 73.) In IPM, chemical pesticides are the strategy of last resort, used only when all other approaches have failed.

Work with community officials to reduce the unnecessary use of pesticides. Encourage communities to adopt IPM policies and to use pest-management staff trained in IPM. After all, what's the point of adopting such a policy if pesticide operators are left to do things the way they see fit?

Once pest policies have shifted to IPM, make sure they stay that way. Many a battle to change over to the least-toxic alternatives for fighting pests is negated when the director of public works sprayer goes back to "business as usual" when no one is paying attention.

86 SMART SOLUTION
Take a stand against road salt.

In the United States, particularly in the North, groundwater (and thus drinking water) can be contaminated by the excessive use of road salt on icy streets. Too much salt in our drinking water is a health hazard, particularly to people with high blood pressure or kidney disease. Growing children also need good drinking water, uncontaminated with excessive runoff from road salt.

☆
Good Idea

△△
Moderately Easy

Work with your community leaders to develop reasonable ways of addressing road hazards due to ice. Encourage them to use more sand and less salt on side streets and to minimize the use of salts whenever possible on major roadways. (In addition to posing a health hazard in the drinking water, road salt is also damaging to trees and shrubs along the highway.)

87 SMART SOLUTION
Support lead paint removal efforts.

Lead paint was used on the exterior and interior of buildings through the 1970s. Its flaking and peeling cause the majority of cases of childhood lead poisoning in the United States.

☆☆☆
Very
Important

Removing old lead paint from buildings is the only sure way to stop generations of children from developing lead poisoning. Support the removal of lead paint from older buildings so that your children and grandchildren don't end up with lead poisoning. (See Smart Solutions 19 – 28 for a detailed description of lead poisoning and how to prevent it.) This issue is being tackled nationwide on government-subsidized housing through an initiative of the United States Department of Housing and Urban Development (HUD). The agency makes funds available to assist with lead-removal projects for its Section 8 housing units (housing units made available for low-income residents). It also requires that landlords who wish to offer subsidized housing to low-income residents under HUD Section 8 do lead paint abatement in those units before children are allowed to occupy them.

△△
Moderately
Easy

This initiative is a good example for your local community to follow. Many communities throughout the country are enacting legislation requiring that those selling houses must disclose any known lead hazards to the potential purchaser. By encouraging this type of legislation in your community—or better yet, by encouraging that lead paint hazards be abated prior to the sale of the house—you can make a difference in childhood lead poisoning.

88 SMART SOLUTION
Support sewage treatment plant improvements.

Our rivers, lakes, and oceans have been the dumping ground for sewage and industrial effluents (wastes) for far too long. Once thought to have an infinite ability to absorb these materials, these bodies of water are changing. Fish populations are diminishing in oceans worldwide, in part due to changes in the balance of nature and in part to pollution. For example, Long Island Sound, which borders New York City, New York State, and Connecticut, receives millions of gallons per day of sewage treatment plant effluent containing nitrogen and phosphorous. Every few years, fish kills are reported as the oxygen levels in the Sound drop so low that fish can't live. How does that happen, you ask?

☆☆
Important

△△
Moderately
Easy

FISH AND PFISTERIA

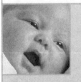 IN NORTH Carolina and in the Chesapeake Bay, a new problem has emerged during the last few years. Fish have become infested with a parasite called pfisteria, resulting in ulcers and considerable bodily damage to the fish. Fishermen in the area have complained that they, too, are experiencing rashes and illness attributed to a toxin produced by the pfisteria. Researchers have noted that the problem seems to occur in areas where excessive nutrients from hog farms (i.e., hog waste runoff that contains nitrogen and phosphorous) are washing into the coastal area inhabited by the fish. This is just another example of how the balance of nature has been subtly altered, creating a new plague that is affecting both man and animals.

Well, the nitrogen and phosphorous deposited into our coastal waters by sewage treatment plants and by runoff from farms, lawns, and gardens encourage the growth of algae, resulting in algae blooms (overproduction of algae). When the algae die, their decomposition uses up the oxygen in the water. Obviously, fish can't survive without oxygen in the water, and they die as a result.

New technology does exist, however, that enables sewage treatment plants to reduce the nitrogen and phosphorous content of sewage effluent. This new technology is expensive, though, and many groups are working to avoid putting it into use—making it even more important that you support such improvements.

89 SMART SOLUTION
Urge a ban on utility-pole preservatives.

Those wooden utility poles that are crucial for carrying electricity to your home also carry a hidden poison: pentachlorophenol. Pentachlorophenol (also known as penta) is a highly toxic chemical that's used to preserve the poles so they can stand up for years without rotting.

Important

Difficult

However, long-term exposure to penta can result in an impaired immune system, reproductive problems, birth defects, cancer, and other health problems. The National Coalition against the Misuse of Pesticides has called for the Environmental Protection Agency to ban all uses of penta. (It's already banned in 26 countries.) And so should you.

If you think your child can't possibly be exposed to penta because she doesn't have much contact with wooden utility poles, think about this: Out of 197 children in Arkansas between the ages of 2 and 6 years who were randomly tested for penta, 197 of them—that's right, *all* of them—had traces of it in their urine.

To learn more about penta and its effects, go to www. beyondpesticides.org.

90

SMART SOLUTION
Work with your elected officials.

Solutions to environmental hazards often lead directly to the door of an elected official. When you contact your elected officials, have a good definition of the problem and, when possible, a proposed solution. Let those in office—at the local, county, state, and federal levels—know that other voters see things the same way that you do. Tell them that a neighborhood association is working on the issue.

☆☆
Important

△△
Moderately
Easy

Elected officials understand that their lifeline is voter satisfaction, so make fixing the problem in their best interest. A "win-win" situation is what you want. The elected official who satisfies the concerns of a community group is in a great position for reelection.

Know which elected official has the greatest chance of solving your problem. For local issues, contact your mayor or city councilman. For issues under the jurisdiction of the state, contact your state legislator and/or governor. For federal issues, contact your congressperson or senator.

Pay attention to the track record of those in political office. Appeal both to those who share your concerns and also to those who need to become better educated on the issue so that they see things from your point of view. Bipartisan coalitions are best and can most effectively be achieved by education of officials. Also find out what environmental issues your elected officials are working on and support them when they meet the needs of the community.

Keep up an ongoing dialogue with elected officials so that the environmental needs of your community get the attention they deserve. Let your elected officials know that you are willing to help in any way with one or more issues they consider important. (For more on specific organizations working to improve the environment, see "Resources" on page 145.)

PART THREE

PROTECTING YOUR FUTURE
CHILDREN

**An Environmental Checklist
for Future Moms and Dads...** *127*

**11 Ways to Protect Parents
from Reproductive Risks...** *130*

AN ENVIRONMENTAL CHECKLIST FOR FUTURE MOMS AND DADS

Planning to have a baby is one of the most exciting times in a person's life. When you think about becoming a parent, you can probably already hear the pitter-patter of tiny feet and feel those little arms wrapped around you in a big hug. Of course, your baby will be your most precious gift, but you, in turn, can give your baby something precious as well—a healthy parent.

That's why limiting your exposure to environmental toxins as much as you can before you start trying to conceive is so important. And although you may feel healthy, environmental hazards at home and at work might be compromising your health.

To find out about potential dangers from environmental hazards, read through this checklist, answering the questions as you go. As you answer, check the numbers (if any) that follow your responses. Those numbers correspond to the numbered "Smart Solutions" throughout this book that can help you prevent or eliminate the unsafe situation.

IN YOUR HOUSE

The boxed numbers indicate which SMART SOLUTION(s) you should review.

Are you RENOVATING your house?
○ Yes 99 100   ○ No

Do you keep cleaners, strippers, and CHEMICALS around your house?
○ Yes 96 100   ○ No

Do you use PESTICIDES around your house?
○ Yes 92   ○ No

(continued)

The boxed numbers indicate which SMART SOLUTION(s) you should review.

Do you have your own household PAINTING, floor REFINISHING, furniture refinishing, or automobile RESTORATION or detail painting business?
○ Yes 91 97   ○ No

Do you use DRUGS or ALCOHOL?
○ Yes 101   ○ No

Do you take prescription MEDICATIONS?
○ Yes 101   ○ No

Are you a SMOKER?
○ Yes 101   ○ No

AT WORK

Do you use OSHA-approved PROTECTIVE clothing and respiratory equipment when required?
○ Yes   ○ No 91

Do you work in a PRINT SHOP?
○ Yes 91   ○ No

Do you work in an INDUSTRIAL or MANUFACTURING firm?
○ Yes 91   ○ No

Do you work in the PETROCHEMICAL industry?
○ Yes 91   ○ No

Do you work with SPRAY PAINTS?
○ Yes 91   ○ No

Do you work in a GAS station or automobile repair shop?
○ Yes 91   ○ No

Is part of your job to replace worn-out BRAKES?
○ Yes 91   ○ No

Does your gas station have adequate EXHAUST systems for fumes?
○ Yes   ○ No 91

Are you exposed to ANTIFREEZE and petroleum product spills that are not immediately cleaned up?
○ Yes 91   ○ No

Do you work in a health clinic, HOSPITAL, or physician's office?
○ Yes 91   ○ No

Are you an X-RAY technician or do you work around an x-ray machine?
○ Yes 91   ○ No

Do you work in an OPERATING ROOM?
○ Yes 91   ○ No

Do you work in a hospital LABORATORY?
○ Yes 91   ○ No

Do you spend time in an enclosed room with a COPY MACHINE?
○ Yes 91   ○ No

Do you work with SPRAY adhesives, fixatives, or rubber cement?
○ Yes 91 97   ○ No

Do you work on a FARM?
○ Yes 91 92   ○ No

Do you know what kinds of PESTICIDES are used on the farm?
○ Yes   ○ No 91 92

Are you a house PAINTER?
○ Yes 91   ○ No

Do you use respiratory PROTECTION when painting indoors?
○ Yes   ○ No 91

Do you use paints with MERCURY or CADMIUM in them?
○ Yes 91   ○ No

Do you use a HEAT GUN to remove paint?
○ Yes 91   ○ No

Do you work in the BUILDING trades?
○ Yes 96   ○ No

Are you a WELDER?
○ Yes 91 93   ○ No

Are you a furniture REFINISHER?
○ Yes 91   ○ No

Do you work in the LEAD industry?
○ Yes 91   ○ No

Have you melted down old BATTERIES?
○ Yes 91   ○ No

Do you work with MERCURY?
○ Yes 91   ○ No

Do you like to go FISHING?
○ Yes 98   ○ No

Do you EAT what you catch?
○ Yes 98   ○ No

YOUR HOBBIES

Do you work with STAINED GLASS?
○ Yes 97   ○ No

Do you do DECOUPAGE?
○ Yes 97   ○ No

Do you restore FURNITURE?
○ Yes 97   ○ No

Do you work with decorative CRAFTS?
○ Yes 97   ○ No

Do you restore old AUTOMOBILES?
○ Yes 96 97   ○ No

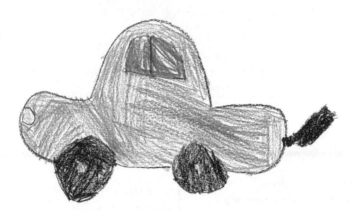

11 Ways to Protect Parents from Reproductive Risks

PROTECTING YOUR child from environmental hazards starts even before your baby is conceived: Healthy babies begin with healthy moms and dads. So to give your baby the best start in life, both of you—mom and dad—need to protect yourselves from environmental hazards that could affect your general health and your reproductive systems. Here are some tips to help you avoid dangerous toxins at work and in your home.

91 SMART SOLUTION
Know what chemical hazards you're being exposed to at work.

If you haven't already read through "An Environmental Checklist for Future Moms and Dads" on page 127, turn back and read it now. This checklist will help you identify some potential health hazards that may exist both in and outside your workplace.

☆☆☆
Very Important

△△△
Difficult

Under Occupational Safety and Health Administration (OSHA) standards and the Environmental Protection Agency (EPA) Right-to-Know Law, you're entitled to know what chemical hazards you're exposed to at work. Your employer is required to maintain material safety data sheets that list the names of any chemicals you work with—and their risks. If an occupational health clinic or an industrial hygienist is present where you work, ask for the data sheets for chemicals or materials used in your workplace.

Here are some chemicals that are known or suspected reproductive hazards—where they're used, the specific problems they cause, and what you can do to avoid reproductive problems from them.

Lead

Lead is a soft, malleable mineral obtained by smelting from quarried rock. Environmental exposure to high levels of lead can cause infertility in men. Pregnant women exposed to high levels of lead can miscarry. Babies born from mothers exposed to high levels of lead may develop neurological problems, experience developmental delays, and have behavioral abnormalities.

Lead is everywhere. Over the years, it has been used in plumbing, paints, and batteries. You can find it in pottery, stained-glass framing, and under the ceramic finish of some pots and pans. Up until the 1970s, lead was added to gasoline to enhance automobile performance and prevent engine knocking; it was also used in solder.

One of the most dangerous workplace exposures to lead comes from lead smelting. The mining and smelting of ore (primary smelting) can poison workers and whole neighborhoods. In Coeur d'Alene, Idaho, for example, a pristine valley between the peaks of the Rockies, a primary lead smelter released 35.3 metric tons of lead emissions into the community in 1974, which resulted in the lead poisoning of 99 percent of the children living within a mile of the plant. The smelter was ultimately closed because of the severe lead poisoning of the community.

Secondary lead smelting can also represent a dangerous workplace exposure. Secondary smelting refers to the reuse of lead by melting down old lead batteries or lead pipes for their lead content. The lead fumes produced by the melting process are readily absorbed by the body and can cause life-threatening consequences.

Painters, contractors, and house renovators can become lead poisoned from lead paint on the exterior or interior of the houses if they don't remove the paint correctly. For example, removing lead paint

IF YOU'RE **EXPOSED TO LEAD** AT WORK, SHOWER AND CHANGE CLOTHES BEFORE YOU GO HOME TO AVOID BRINGING LEAD DUST INTO YOUR HOUSE OR CAR AND EXPOSING YOUR FAMILY.

with a heat gun can produce extremely high levels of lead in the blood. Lead vaporizes at a fairly low temperature and creates a fume that is then readily absorbed when inhaled. Sandblasting exterior lead paint can also cause lead poisoning in both workers and community residents.

What to do. If your job requires you to be exposed to lead, make sure to use OSHA-approved safety equipment. (See "Resources" on page 145 for additional information on OSHA regulations.) Also see Smart Solutions [19]–[21] for additional lead-safety information.

Asbestos

Asbestos is a group of fibrous minerals that are used as insulation and for their resistance to heat, acid, and fire. You can find asbestos in homes, schools, and buildings built between the 1920s and the 1970s, after which it was phased out. You can also find asbestos in automobile brakes.

Long-term exposure to asbestos causes lung cancer mesothelioma, a cancer of the lung's lining. (Also see [74] for more information on the health effects of asbestos.) Although asbestos isn't known to be a reproductive health hazard, the health effects it can cause are serious.

If you work in the building trades, you may become exposed to asbestos during demolition and renovation work on older buildings. And automobile repair shop workers can become exposed to asbestos when repairing brakes because asbestos is used in brake linings to retard the buildup of heat.

What to do. Use OSHA-approved safety equipment at work. If you believe that asbestos is being used improperly in your workplace, you have the right to contact OSHA to request an inspection.

Cadmium

Cadmium is a metal used in the manufacture of paints and other industrial processes. The reproductive health effects of cadmium are not completely known at this time. However, many health-care professionals are concerned that exposure to cadmium may cause a pregnant woman to miscarry; there is also concern that it is related to lung development problems in babies, contributing to respiratory distress syndrome. In animals, cadmium damages the male reproductive system and sperm, which leads researchers to believe it may damage a human male's reproductive system, as well.

Cadmium is also a common component of many oil paints. If you're an artist who uses oil paints, your exposure to this metal can be enhanced if you practice "tipping" your brush (putting your brush into your mouth to draw the hairs into a fine tip).

What to do. Use OSHA-approved safety equipment at work. If you're an artist, don't "tip" your brush, and avoid getting any paint containing cadmium on your skin.

Mercury

Mercury is available in several forms, each of which is characterized by a different type of toxicity.

Elemental mercury is a silvery liquid metal that breaks apart into droplets and coalesces into larger pools. It can vaporize at room temperature and enter your body rapidly if you inhale the vapor. Elemental mercury is linked with neurological damage in persons of all ages, but especially in infants and unborn children.

Mercury is used in street and road lighting, as a fungicide in paints, in some fungicides and antiseptics, and in dental fillings. Mercury is also used in thermometers and mercury switches for a wide variety of industrial and commercial purposes, as well as in many batteries. For example, those popular children's sneakers that light up as they walk contain mercury switches.

What to do. Use OSHA-approved safety equipment at work. To prevent mercury poisoning at home, avoid using products containing mercury, such as fungicides and paints. You should also replace your mercury thermometer

CLEANING UP A SPILL

TO CLEAN up a minor mercury spill, such as a broken thermometer, push the beads into a sealable container with a piece of cardboard—*don't* touch the mercury. Seal the container, then call your local health department to find out where to discard it. Don't use a vacuum to try to suck up the mercury because the vacuum will vaporize the mercury and you could potentially inhale the vapors.

Do *not* attempt to clean up a mercury spill that's larger than the spill from a broken thermometer. Let professionals handle any spills larger than that. Call your local or state health department for assistance with household or neighborhood spills, and call OSHA for assistance with spills at work.

with a digital one. Keep mercury out of landfills (and help prevent problems for future generations of children) by recycling batteries instead of throwing them in the trash. Those sneakers with mercury switches are a problem at landfills, as well, so buy regular sneakers for your kids.

Glycol Ethers

Glycol ethers are solvents that are used as industrial cleaners. When breathed in, they can cause testicular damage in men. Animal studies show that glycol ethers may also affect the reproductive health of women.

Deicing fluids, pesticides, cosmetics, cleaning solutions, inks, varnishes, paints, circuit boards, and chemicals used in the printing and photography trades are all places where you can find glycol ethers used as solvents. Glycol ethers have also been used as degreasing agents in metal trades, although their use has begun to decline as more people have become aware of their potential for reproductive toxicity.

What to do. If you work with glycol ethers, keep up with developing research by periodically reviewing material safety data sheets on these materials, or by checking with the health and safety department where you work. Use OSHA-approved safety equipment. Also avoid using products containing ethylene glycol whenever possible.

Radiation

Radiation, those invisible waves emitted by x-ray machines and industrial radiation sources, is very hazardous. Exposure to radiation can damage the reproductive system in both men and women and can cause cancer. X-ray technicians and people who work in facilities that use radioactive equipment are at risk for exposure.

What to do. Use OSHA-approved safety equipment at work. Use dosimeters (devices used for measuring radiation) and workplace safety standards without fail. If you're pregnant, you need to be especially careful around all types of radiation because the fetus is more sensitive to radiation than adults. When in doubt, check with your doctor.

Solvents

Solvents are used in various industries in degreasers, paints, varnishes, paint removers, dry-cleaning agents, printing and copier chemicals, and laboratory chemicals. They are also used in hair salons for gluing on false fingernails. One solvent, benzene, is known to cause cancer and has been linked with leukemia in people who work with it. Benzene and other solvents, such as trichlorethylene and perchlorethylene, have also been linked with causing reproductive problems in men and women. And several studies have shown the solvent toluene to cause birth defects and miscarriage.

What to do. Use OSHA-approved safety equipment at work. Avoid the use of benzene and benzene-containing solvents whenever possible, as well as chlorinated solvents like methylene chloride. If you work in a hair or nail salon, make sure you work in a well-ventilated area.

At home, wear appropriate respiratory equipment such as a proper chemical respirator with fresh cartridges (not just a little dust mask), and always work outdoors when using solvents or degreasers.

Anesthetic Gases

Some gases used for anesthesia, especially halothane, cause reproductive problems. In fact, nurses who work in the operating room have been shown to have a high risk of miscarriage. We advise pregnant women to minimize occupational exposure to all types of anesthesia.

What to do. If you work in an operating room, be sure that the most recent technology for anesthetic gas recovery in is place so that your exposure to the gases is minimal.

Also, if you're pregnant or intending to become pregnant, discuss your exposure to anesthetic gases in the operating room with your obstetrician/gynecologist to find out if he thinks you should limit your exposure during pregnancy.

92
SMART SOLUTION
Avoid exposure to pesticides, PCBs, and other chlorinated hydrocarbons.

A growing body of data shows that some pesticides, polychlorinated biphenyls (PCBs), and related chemicals (chlorinated hydrocarbons) have the ability to interfere with the normal functioning of hormones. Known as endocrine disrupters, these chemicals mimic the normal functioning of hormones, including estrogen and thyroid hormones.

☆☆☆
Very
Important

△△
Moderately
Easy

Some chlorinated hydrocarbons associated with possible reproductive problems include epichlorhydrin (a powerful reproductive toxin in animals) and ethylene dibromide (a fumigant used in grains). Ethylene oxide, a nonchlorinated compound used as a fumigant in hospital operating rooms and elsewhere, has been linked with male infertility. Agent Orange, a defoliant used during the Vietnam War, contained a potent herbicide called 2,4,5-D that produced dioxin. Dioxin is another chemical that fits into the class called "endocrine disrupters." Vietnam veterans attributed birth defects in their children to exposure to Agent Orange; although medical research was not able to confirm this, there's no question that dioxin has the potential to cause reproductive problems.

Laboratory data have shown that the endocrine disrupters have the ability to bind to the sites in the cells where hormones usually go. In theory, even tiny quantities of pesticides in the body may be a problem—and it takes only a minuscule amount of a hormone to set a whole chain of action in motion. So it's possible that endocrine disrupters might compete with normal hormonal functioning, causing havoc in your body or developmental problems in your unborn child or infant.

None of this has been proven in people to date. However, the theory fits observations of what has occurred and continues to occur in wildlife. (See "Dangers of Endocrine Disrupters" on the opposite page.)

It's too early to tell whether the same effects that have occurred in animals can occur in people and what amount of pesticide causes such health problems. However, several instances have been documented where endocrine disrupters caused adverse reproductive effects in people.

Dibromochloropropane (DBCP). This pesticide, used to control insects on fruit crops, was manufactured in a California plant starting in 1962. During the 1970s, a group of young men working in the plant realized that none of them had been able to father children, although in the past some of them had been fertile. In 1976, physicians examined a group of these men, and they found that the men had exceedingly low sperm counts. DBCP was banned in the United States in the 1970s after studies indicated that men exposed to the pesticide at work became sterile.

Diethylstilbesterol (DES). This chemical mimics estrogen. From the 1950s through 1971, DES was considered a wonder drug that could help women at risk of miscarriage

DANGERS OF ENDOCRINE DISRUPTERS

DECADES AGO, in her book *Silent Spring*, Rachel Carson linked the vanishing populations of eagles to the widespread use of a chlorinated hydrocarbon pesticide, DDT (dichlorodiphenyltrichloroethane). DDT was banned in this country for use on food crops in the early 1970s and was banned for all other uses by the late 1980s. DDT interfered with the reproduction of birds by making their eggshells too soft to withstand the incubation and hatching process. Considered a wonder drug in the 1940s when malaria was rampant, DDT was sprayed with abandon in communities to thwart the mosquitoes that carry the malaria parasite. A TV news crew of the time captured the spraying of crowds of children at Long Island swimming pools with DDT. It was rebroadcast in 1998 by New York City media—at a time when the elevated rate of breast cancer in Long Island women was being investigated by area researchers.

In the 1980s, a spill of dicofol (a pesticide) contaminated with DDT in Lake Apopka, Florida, was linked to alligators born with abnormal reproductive organs, mixed gender alligators, and unusually high death rates for the hatchlings.

Other wildlife and animal laboratory studies have shown reproductive problems related to pesticides that are used to spray fruits and vegetables, trees, lawns, and ornamental shrubbery. These pesticides include methoxychlor, endosulfan, lindane, dicofol, vinclozolin, and cypermethrin.

carry their baby to full term. In 1970, a cluster of young women whose mothers had taken DES while pregnant developed unusual types of vaginal cancer—which, in turn, alerted the medical community to the dangers of DES. These young women later experienced reduced fertility and other reproductive problems. DES was also found to cause reproductive abnormalities in some male babies exposed in utero to the drug.

Hypospadias. Over the past several decades, an epidemic of hypospadias, a male reproductive birth defect in which the opening of the penis is located on the underside rather than the tip, has occurred. (This condition has increased not just in the United States but worldwide.) The Centers for Disease Control and Prevention has reported a doubling of this condition during the past two decades in a seven-county area around Atlanta that is used to monitor birth defects. Some researchers are concerned that these increases may correlate with the enormous increase of endocrine disrupters and hormone mimics in our society over the past several decades. Again, although no data currently exist to support or reject this hypothesis, pediatricians and health scientists are becoming increasingly concerned that these reproductive problems may be linked to exposure to endocrine disrupters.

What to do. Use OSHA-approved safety equipment at work. If you're a landscaper, pesticide applicator, or plant nursery worker, check with your local cooperative extension office for courses in Integrated Pest Management (IPM) and using the least-toxic alternatives to do the job. Phase out the use of the most toxic materials and substitute organic and less-toxic alternatives to accomplish the task.

If your job requires that you work with pesticides, see your physician or an occupational health clinic to make sure the chemicals aren't adversely affecting your health. If you have concerns that your needs aren't being addressed by your employer or on-site employee health facility, see "Resources" on page 145 for a nationwide listing of independent occupational health centers.

At home, avoid using pesticides. Nontoxic alternatives are available for virtually every common pest problem. Check with your local cooperative extension office for information on IPM and for suggestions regarding the least-toxic alternative to solve your problem. Another source of information is Beyond Pesticides/NCAMP (National Coalition against the Misuse of Pesticides; see "Resources" on page 145).

93 SMART SOLUTION
Practice safe welding.

Welding is related to a host of health issues, including respiratory problems and cancer. In addition, some studies have shown reproductive problems (infertility) related to welding, especially stainless steel welding. These health problems appear to be caused by inhaling the toxic fumes that are produced when welding.

Important

Easy

If you're a welder or welding is part of your job, make sure you wear OSHA-approved safety equipment while welding and make sure that you're working in a properly ventilated space.

94
Avoid tobacco smoke.

Tobacco smoke is known to cause cancer, and the chemicals in tobacco smoke can damage the reproductive system in both men and women. And tobacco smoking has been linked with impotence.

☆☆☆
Very Important

If you smoke, now is the time to stop. (See Smart Solution ⑮ for other reasons to stop and helpful hints on how to do it.) Don't let people smoke in your house. If your workplace isn't smoke free, work to have it declared so.

△△△
Difficult

Also find out what your local laws say about smoking in public places, and work with community groups to increase the number of smoke-free places in your community. (See ⑧①)

95
Provide an occupational history.

Your exposure to various workplace chemicals and hazardous materials over the years can cause health problems. Unless your physician knows what you've been exposed to, he may not be able to advise you what to do to protect your health. If your industry has an occupational health clinic or an industrial hygienist, ask for exposure data or health information sheets applicable to your workplace and give these to your physician.

☆☆
Important

△
Easy

Many physicians routinely ask for occupational histories from their patients. If yours hasn't taken your occupational history, bring a form along to your next appointment and ask him to do so. (Contact OSHA for information on obtaining an occupational history form; see "Resources" on page 145.)

96
Get rid of the big 3.

Lead paint, radon, and asbestos can present huge dangers to your own health, as well as to the health of any children you have. Lead paint, for example, can put you at risk for reproductive problems if it's removed from your house the wrong way. And as we've said repeatedly throughout this book, lead paint is the cause of most childhood poisonings. (See Smart Solutions ⑲–㉒ ㉔) And both asbestos and radon contribute to lung cancer. (See ㊕㊖) So you can see why it's very important that your home is free of these major toxins.

☆☆☆
Very Important

△△
Moderately Easy

97

SMART SOLUTION
Pursue hobbies safely.

The materials involved in some hobbies such as furniture stripping and oil painting can be hazardous to your health—turning a fun activity into dangerous one.

☆☆
Important

△△
Moderately
Easy

That doesn't mean you have to give up your hobby, though—you just need to be aware of the hazards and use some safe practices. Here's what you need to know.

Furniture stripping. Avoid using strippers that contain methylene chloride, a toxic solvent that has been linked with serious health problems such as blood disorders and heart attacks. (See Smart Solution 17) And make sure you do your furniture stripping outdoors, where you'll get the best possible ventilation.

Stained glass. The solder and camber used in making stained glass pieces may be made of lead. Use non-lead solder and camber to avoid causing lead poisoning in yourself and your family.

Oil painting. If you paint, the paints and solvents (such as turpentine) that you use contain many toxic materials, including lead, cadmium, and other heavy metals. To prevent exposure to the toxins in oil paints, don't tip your brush (put it into your mouth to draw the bristles together)—and don't smoke while painting, which can increase the risk of transmitting the paint from your hands to your mouth (in addition to being a fire hazard).

If you work in an enclosed area, the concentration of turpentine can reach unacceptably high levels, causing headaches, dizziness, and other symptoms of nervous system toxicity. Your best bet here is to use alternatives to turpentine and also, of course, to use good ventilation. Try using artist's oils to clean your brushes between strokes of paint. If paint gets on your skin, remove it with Avon's Skin-So-Soft, which contains light oils and emulsifiers.

Decorative crafts. Paints, glues, and solvents used in craft making, including decoupage, model airplane and car crafts, and doll house making, can be hazardous to your health. (See 91) Make sure you work in a well-ventilated room, take frequent breaks, and avoid using products containing toxic chemicals.

Automobile repair and restoration. Paints and fumes from solvents can be hazardous to your health. (See 91) Make sure you always work in a well-ventilated area and take frequent breaks.

AVOID THESE FISH

IF YOU'RE planning to conceive (or if you're already pregnant), avoid eating shark, swordfish, king mackerel, and tile fish because they could contain high levels of mercury, according to the Food and Drug Administration. Mercury ingested during pregnancy can damage an unborn baby's central nervous system, leaving the baby with slower than normal brain development.

98 SMART SOLUTION
Choose fresh fish wisely.

The taste of a freshly caught fish sure beats a frozen fillet from a grocery store any day. What you can't taste in fish, though, are contaminants they may have ingested, such as PCBs (polychlorinated biphenyls). (See Smart Solution 41) As we mentioned earlier in the book, many of our pristine trout streams and estuaries are contaminated by PCBs and other toxins. Even ocean fish, such as swordfish, aren't immune to toxins that accumulate in the water.

☆☆
Important

△△
Moderately Easy

So how can you enjoy eating local fish safely?

- Find out which water bodies in your area are contaminated (contact your state health department for a list). Don't eat more than the recommended amount of each type of fish from water bodies that are contaminated. If both eels and bluefish are listed as fish that you're not supposed to eat more than once a week, eat one or the other, not both, during the same week.

- Vary the sources of the fish you eat.

- Avoid eating the fatty areas on fish, which is where the toxins accumulate.

99 SMART SOLUTION
Time household renovations.

Once you start to think about having a baby, you may realize that you need to do some renovations around your home. (See Smart Solution 1) Perhaps you need to turn your room into the baby's room. Or maybe you want to enlarge your kitchen because you'll certainly need the extra space.

☆☆
Important

△△
Moderately Easy

However, renovating your house (or having someone else do it) while you're planning a pregnancy or once you're already pregnant may expose you to toxic chemicals, depending on what's being renovated. A lead-poisoned father-to-be may not be able to have children. Lead poisoning in the mother-to-be can be very dangerous for the baby because lead can cross the placenta and injure the child. During pregnancy, the mother's bones mobilize (rearrange on a microscopic level) to provide minerals for the developing baby's bones. If the mother's bones contain lead from a previous bout of lead poisoning, some of that lead will move into the baby and the baby's bones will contain some lead, too. If the mother is lead poisoned during pregnancy, the lead will find itself in the baby's developing nervous system.

So, keep out of harm's way. Do any household renovation projects well before baby is conceived. If that's not possible, make sure the pregnant mom relocates to another house while potentially dangerous lead dust and toxic solvents are being generated during the renovation. If dad is involved in the renovation work, make sure he uses appropriate protective equipment and follows the safety guidelines for the project to the letter of the law.

100

SMART SOLUTION
Reduce using chemicals in your home.

Society dictates that we have ultraclean, germ-free, pristine homes. And to accomplish that, of course, we supposedly need a huge amount of chemical products in our arsenal. You may be surprised to learn, though, just how many household chemicals you can do without. Try this 4-week plan.

☆☆
Important

△
Easy

Week 1. List all the cleaning supplies in your house (don't forget those under your kitchen sink). Cross off all but the five you consider most useful. This week, use only those household chemicals you've listed as most important. Keep a record of what you really needed and couldn't use because it wasn't on your list.

Week 2. Add up to two more household chemicals that you wish you had on your list during that first week. Move the chemicals you're not using to a more inaccessible area of your house: a box in the basement or garden storage area.

Week 3. Donate all unnecessary household chemicals to the next household chemical clean-up day in your community. (See Smart Solution 52)

Week 4. Now that you've weaned yourself from the plethora of marble cleaners and venetian blind concoctions, take a good look at the list of ingredients on the containers of the seven household chemicals you've decided to use. Consider replacing each product with a less-toxic version of the same item. Check your grocery store and "Resources" on page 145 for sources of less-toxic household cleaning products. When you absolutely need to use a chemical for cleaning, buy the product in the smallest quantity available, and use it up rather than store it.

101 SMART SOLUTION
Avoid using tobacco, alcohol, and illicit drugs during pregnancy.

Very Important

If you're already pregnant or are planning to become pregnant in the near future, you need to pay special attention to this information. As a future mom, protecting your unborn baby's health is your responsibility.

Don't smoke during pregnancy. Tobacco smoke can cause △△△ **Difficult** premature delivery and low-birthweight babies. While quitting before you become pregnant is ideal, kicking the tobacco habit while you're pregnant will still help your baby's health. Ask your doctor for help in quitting, as well as for a list of local support groups for smokers trying to stop.

Avoiding alcohol while you're pregnant is just as important as not smoking. Babies of mothers who used alcohol to excess during pregnancy can have fetal alcohol syndrome. This is a very severe birth defect that causes facial abnormalities and mental retardation.

And as far as illicit drugs are concerned, simply remember this: What goes into your body goes into your baby's body. If you use marijuana, cocaine, or any other type of illicit drug during your pregnancy, your baby is using that drug, too. Check with your doctor or pharmacist before taking any over-the-counter and prescription drugs as well.

With this last Smart Solution, we've brought our book back full circle to where we started with the first Smart Solution—planning for a new baby.

We hope that you'll refer to these pages not just while your baby is an infant, but time and again as your children grow and as you move into new homes and neighborhoods. After all, bringing up healthy children is a challenge in our world of toxins. But we know you can do it. A healthy environment is one of the best gifts you can give your children—and a priceless legacy for your children's children, as well.

Recommended Reading

General Reference

Berman, Alan. *Your Naturally Healthy Home: Stylish, Safe, Simple.* Emmaus, PA: Rodale, 2001.

Bhagat, S. *Your Health and the Environment: A Study/Action Guide for Congregations.* New York: Eco-Justice Working Group, National Council of Churches of Christ in the USA, 1998.

Needleman, Herbert L., M.D., and Philip J. Landrigan, M.D. *Raising Children Toxic Free.* New York: Morrow/Avon, 1995.

Pennybacker, Mindy, and Aisha Ikramuddin. *Guide to Natural Baby Care.* New York: John Wiley & Sons, 1999.

Schultz, Warren. *The Organic Suburbanite: An Environmentally Friendly Way to Live the American Dream.* Emmaus, PA: Rodale, 2001.

Van Straten, Michael. *Organic Living.* Emmaus, PA: Rodale, 2001.

Community Organizing

Pick, Maritza. *How to Save Your Neighborhood, City, or Town.* San Francisco: Sierra Club Books, 1993.

Household Cleaners

Berthold-Bond, Annie. *Better Basics for the Home.* Toronto: Crown Publishing Group, 1999.

———. *Clean and Green.* Woodstock, NY: Ceres Press, 1994.

Organic Foods

Berthold-Bond, Annie, et al. *Green Kitchen Handbook.* New York: Harper Trade, 1997.

Vann, Lizzie. *Organic Baby and Toddler Cookbook: Easy Recipes for Natural Food.* New York: DK Publishing, 2001.

Organic Gardening

Bradley, Fern Marshall, and Barbara W. Ellis, eds. *Rodale's All-New Encyclopedia of Organic Gardening.* Emmaus, PA: Rodale, 1992.

Bucks, Christine, ed. *Rodale Organic Gardening Basics: Perennials.* Emmaus, PA: Rodale, 2001.

Bucks, Christine, ed. *Rodale Organic Gardening Basics: Pests.* Emmaus, PA: Rodale, 2001.

Bucks, Christine, ed. *Rodale Organic Gardening Basics: Vegetables.* Emmaus, PA: Rodale, 2000.

Soltys, Karen Costello, ed. *Rodale Organic Gardening Basics: Lawns.* Emmaus, PA: Rodale, 2000.

Newsletters and Magazines

Beyond Pesticides
701 E Street SE
Suite 200
Washington, DC 20003
Web site: www.beyondpesticides.org
Newsletter of the National Coalition against the Misuse of Pesticides

Common Sense Pest Quarterly
P.O. Box 7414
Berkley, CA 94707
Web site: www.birc.org
Quarterly journal of the Bio-Integral Resource Center

Consumer Reports
Consumers Union
101 Truman Avenue
Yonkers, New York 10703
Web site: www.consumerreports.org

OG
Rodale, Inc.
33 East Minor Street
Emmaus, PA 18098
Web site: www.organicgardening.com

Resources

General Information

Alliance to End Childhood Lead Poisoning
227 Massachusetts Avenue NE
Suite 200
Washington, DC 20002
Phone: (202) 543-1147
E-mail: aeclp@aeclp.org
Web site: www.aeclp.org
Nonprofit dedicated to preventing childhood lead poisoning; provides information and resources

The Association of Occupational & Environmental Clinics
1010 Vermont Avenue NW
#513
Washington, DC 20005
Phone: (202) 347-4956
E-mail: aoec@aoec.org
Web site: www.aoec.org
Nonprofit organization working to improve occupational and environmental health; Web site provides nationwide listing of member clinics

Beyond Pesticides/National Coalition against the Misuse of Pesticides
701 E Street SE
Suite 200
Washington, DC 20003
Phone: (202) 543-5450
E-mail: info@beyondpesticides.org
Web site: beyondpesticides.org
Nonprofit organization committed to adoption of alternative pesticide strategies; publishes two newsletters and other publications

Children's Health Environmental Coalition (CHEC)
P.O. Box 1540
Princeton, NJ 08542
Phone: (609) 252-1915
E-mail: chec@checnet.org
Web site: www.checnet.org
Nonprofit research organization that examines causes of childhood cancers

New York State Occupational Health Clinic Network
Phone: (800) 458-1158 (New York State Department of Health)
Web site: www.health.state.ny.us/nysdoh/environ/occupate.htm
New York State's clinics for diagnosis and prevention of occupational disease

U.S. Department of Labor
OSHA
Office of Public Affairs
Room N3647
200 Constitution Avenue
Washington, DC 20210
Phone: (202) 693-1999
Web site: www.osha.gov
U.S. governmental agency regulating safety and health standards in the workplace; information on lead standards

U.S. Environmental Protection Agency
Office of the Administrator
Office of Children's Health Protection
1200 Pennsylvania Avenue NW
Mail Code 1107A
Washington, DC 20004
Phone: (202) 564-2188
E-mail: www.epa.gov/children/comments.htm
Web site: www.epa.gov/children/whowe/contact.htm
U.S. governmental agency office on children's health issues, including drinking water, air pollution, neurotoxic substances

Asthma and Allergies

Allergy Control Products, Inc.
96 Danbury Road
Ridgefield, CT 06877
Phone: (800) 422-3878
Web site: www.allergycontrol.com
Air filters; allergy-friendly vacuum-cleaner bags; cotton/polyester barrier-cloth fabric

Allergy Resources
3920 Wadsworth Boulevard
Wheatridge, CO 80033
Phone: (800) 873-3529
Web site: www.allergyresources.com
HEPA filters; organic cotton mattresses and encasements; pillows and sheets

Allergy Solutions, Inc.
7 Crozerville Road
Aston, PA 19014
Phone: (800) 491-4300
Web site: www.allergysolution.com
Dust-mite-proof bedding; air purifiers; HEPA vacuum cleaners; scent-free cleaning products

American Environmental Health Foundation
8345 Walnut Hill Lane
Suite 225
Dallas, TX 75231
Phone: (800) 428-2343
Web site: www.aehf.com
HEPA air filters and purifiers

Breathefree.com, Inc.
12661 Hidden Creek Way
Suite E
Cerritos, CA 90703
Phone: (888) 434-8313
Web site: www.breathefree.com
HEPA filter vacuums; freestanding humidifiers; humidifiers that attach to furnaces; electronic air cleaners with HEPA filters

Euroclean
1151 Bryn Mawr Avenue
Itasca, IL 60143
Phone: (800) 545-4372
Web site: www.eurocleanusa.com
HEPA filter vacuums

Real Goods Trading Corp.
360 Interlocken Boulevard
Suite 300
Broomfield, CO 80021-3440
Phone: (800) 762-7325
Web site: www.realgoods.com
Mattress encasements; organic cotton mattresses and pillows; untreated cotton towels and curtains; rugs; HEPA air purifiers

The Soap Factory
3 Burlington Road
Bedford, MA 01730
Phone: (888) 227-8453
Web site: www.alcasoft.com/soapfact/
Handcrafted olive-oil castile soap

Baby Care

Babyworks
11725 NW West Road
Portland, OR 97229
Phone: (800) 422-2910
Web site: www.babyworks.com
Cotton and wool diapers; diaper covers; wipes; untreated blankets; natural-fiber dolls

Ecobaby
332 Coogan Way
El Cajon, CA 92020
Phone: (888) ECO-BABY (320-2129)
Web site: www.ecobaby.com
Furniture; organic cotton bedding, bath towels, toys, and clothing; disposable diapers; silicone nipples; cleaning products

Ecosport
3871 Sweeten Creek Road
Arden, NC 28704
Phone: (828) 232-1904
Web site: www.ecosport.net
Organic cotton clothing, stuffed animals, sheets, and blankets

Eco-wise
110 West Elizabeth Street
Austin, TX 78704
Phone: (512) 326-4474
Web site: www.ecowise.com
Organic/green cotton diapers, pads, and covers; nursing pads; organic cotton clothing, bedding, mattresses, and baby slings; organic baby food

Evenflo
Attn: Feeding Department
1801 Commerce Drive
Piqua, OH 45356
Phone: (800) 233-5921
Web site: www.evenflo.com
Baby bottles; silicone nipples and pacifiers

Natural Baby Company
7835 Freedom Avenue NW
North Canton, OH 44720-6907
Phone: (800) 388-2229
Web site: http://store.yahoo.com/
    naturalbaby/info.html
*Cotton blankets; wool blankets and mattress
pads; organic cotton cothing, diapers, and
covers; cotton changing pads; nursing pads
and bras; olive-oil castile soap; toys;
beeswax crayons*

Solonia, Inc.
195 South 33rd Street
Boulder, CO 80303-3425
Phone: (303) 499-7963
Web site: www.solonia.com
Organic cotton baby clothing

Household Cleaners

Gaiam, Inc.
360 Interlocken Boulevard
Suite 300
Broomfield, CO 80021
Phone: (303) 464-3600
Web site: www.gaiam.com
*Seventh Generation cleaning products;
anti-allergy sprays and powders; HEPA air
filters and vacuums; fans*

Healthy Home Center
1403-A Cleveland Street
Clearwater, FL 33755
Phone: (800) 583-9523
Web site: www.healthyhome.com
*Alternative rug shampoos; paint removers
without methylene chloride; building
materials*

Organic Provisions
P.O. Box 756
Richboro, PA 18954-0756
Phone: (800) 490-0044
Web site: www.orgfood.com
*Ecover cleaning products containing no
petroleum-based detergents, synthetic per-
fume, or coloring*

Seventh Generation, Inc.
212 Battery Street
Suite A
Burlington, VT 05401-5281
Phone: (802) 658-3773
Web site: www.seventhgen.com
Cleaning and household products

Paints

Chem-Safe Products
P.O. Box 33023
San Antonio, TX 78265
Phone: (210) 657-5321
*Manufacturer of paints without VOC or
biocide; call for dealer information*

Duron Paints and Wallcoverings
10406 Tucker Street
Beltsville, MD 20705
Phone: 800-723-8766
Web site: www.duron.com
Genesis Odor-Free no-VOC paint

Eco-Wise
110 West Elizabeth Street
Austin, TX 78704
Phone: 512-326-4474
Web site: www.ecowise.com
*No-VOC, no-fungicide, and low-biocide
paints with natural pigments*

Environmental Home Center
1724 4th Avenue South
Seattle, WA 98134
Phone: (800) 281-9785
Web site: www.built-e.com
*Pesticide-free carpet with natural backing;
flooring; organic cotton mattresses and bedding; cotton shower curtains; air purifiers
and filters, plant-based paint; lumber*

**LIVOS Phytochemistry of America,
Inc.**
P.O. Box 1740
Mashpee, MA 02649
Phone: (508) 477-7955
Web site: livos@livos.com
*Wood finish products and paint remover
made from natural ingredients*

Natural Choice
1365 Rufina Circle
Santa Fe, NM 87505
Phone: (800) 621-2591
Web site: www.bioshieldpaint.com
*Bioshield paint, polish, and cleaning
products that are no- or low-VOC*

Organic Fertilizer, Pest Management Supplies

Avon
Phone: (800) FOR-AVON (367-2866)
Web site: www.avon.com
Makers of Skin-So-Soft

Biocontrol Network
5116 Williamsburg Road
Brentwood, TN 37027
Phone: (800) 441-2847
www.biconet.com
*Suppliers of alternative pest-control
products; nontoxic lice shampoo; biological
termite control*

Gardener's Supply Company
128 Intervale Road
Burlington, VT 05401
Phone: (800) 427-3363
Web site: www.gardeners.com
Organic fertilizers and pest controls

Gardens Alive!
5100 Schenly Place
Lawrenceburg, IN 47025
Phone: (812) 537-8651
Web site: www.gardens-alive.com
*Organic fertilizers and pest controls; corn
gluten for weed control; natural pet-care
products*

Peaceful Valley Farm Supply
P.O. Box 2209
Grass Valley, CA 95945
Phone: (888) 784-1722
Web site: www.groworganic.com
*Organic fertilizers and pest controls; natural
pet-care products*

Radon Tests

First Alert
3901 Liberty Street Road
Aurora, IL 60504
Phone: (800) 323-9005
Web site: www.firstalert.com
Short-term radon tests; smoke detectors

**Key Technology Radon Gas Testing
Products**
P.O. Box 562
Jonestown, PA 17038
Phone: (800) 523-4964
Web site: www.keyradon.com
Radon test kits and analysis

Credits

Index